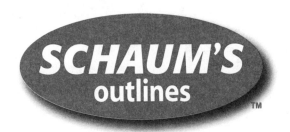

ECG Interpretation

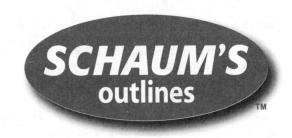

ECG Interpretation

James Keogh, R.N.
Instructor, New York University

Dana Reed, R.N., A.C.N.P., C.C.R.N.
Critical Care Educator, The Valley Hospital

Schaum's Outline Series

New York   Chicago   San Francisco   Lisbon   London   Madrid
Mexico City   Milan   New Delhi   San Juan   Seoul
Singapore   Sydney   Toronto

JIM KEOGH is a registered nurse and has written *Schaum's Outline of Pharmacology, Schaum's Outline of Nursing Laboratory and Diagnostic Tests, Schaum's Outline of Medical Charting,* and co-authored *Schaum's Outline of ECG Interpretation.* His books can be found in leading university libraries, including Yale University School of Medicine, University of Pennsylvania Biomedical Library, Columbia University, Brown University, University of Medicine and Dentistry of New Jersey, Cambridge University, and Oxford University. Jim Keogh, R.N., A.A.S., M.B.A., is a former member of the faculty at Columbia University and is a member of the faculty of New York University.

DANA REED is an acute care nurse practitioner and a nationally certified critical care nurse. He is currently the critical care educator at The Valley Hospital at Ridgewood. He has been on the board of directors for the Northern New Jersey American Association of Critical Care Nurses and is currently the treasurer for the Bergen-Passaic Nurse Educators, a local affiliate of the NNSDO.

Schaum's Outline of
ECG INTERPRETATION

1 2 3 4 5 6 7 8 9 10   QDB / QDB   1 9 8 7 6 5 4 3 2 1

ISBN   978-0-07-173648-0 (print book)
MHID   0-07-173648-4

ISBN   978-0-07-173649-7 (e-book)
MHID   0-07-173649-2

This publication is designed to provide accurate and authoritative information in regard to the subject matter covered. It is sold with the understanding that neither the author nor the publisher is engaged in rendering legal, accounting, securities trading, or other professional services. If legal advice or other expert assistance is required, the services of a competent professional person should be sought.

—From a Declaration of Principles Jointly Adopted by a Committee of the American Bar Association and a Committee of Publishers and Associations

Library of Congress Cataloging-in-Publication Data

Keogh, James, 1948- author.
  Schaum's outline of ECG interpretation / James Keogh, R.N., Instructor, New York University, Dana Reed, R.N., Critical Care Educator, Valley Hospital.
    p. ; cm. — (Schaum's outline series)
  Outline of ECG interpretation
  Summary: "This book provides a review for ECG Interpretation for nursing students"—Provided by publisher.
  ISBN-13: 978-0-07-173648-0 (pbk. : acid-free paper)
  ISBN-10: 0-07-173648-4 (pbk. : acid-free paper)
  ISBN-13: 978-0-07-173649-7 (e-book)
  ISBN-10: 0-07-173649-2 (e-book)
  1. Electrocardiography—Interpretation—Examinations, questions, etc.   2. Electrocardiography—Interpretation—Outlines, syllabi, etc.   3. Heart—Diseases—Diagnosis—Examinations, questions, etc.   4. Heart—Diseases—Diagnosis—Outlines, syllabi, etc.   I. Reed, Dana, author. II. Title. III. Title: Outline of ECG interpretation.
  [DNLM: 1. Electrocardiography—nursing—Examination Questions. 2. Electrocardiography—nursing—Outlines. 3. Heart Diseases—diagnosis—Examination Questions.
  4. Heart Diseases—diagnosis—Outlines. WG 18.2]

RC683.5.E5K462 2011
616.1'207547—dc22   2010047022

McGraw-Hill books are available at special quantity discounts to use as premiums and sales promotions, or for use in corporate training programs. To contact a representative please e-mail us at bulksales@mcgraw-hill.com.

This book is dedicated to Anne, Sandy, Joanne, Amber-Leigh Christine, Shawn, Eric, and Amy, without whose help and support this book couldn't have been written.

James Keogh

To my wife and very best friend, Debbie. And to my two biggest fans and little men, John and James.

Dana Reed

Contents

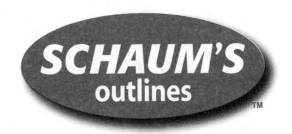

ECG Interpretation

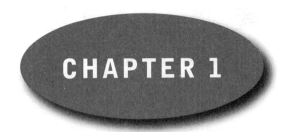
Anatomy and Physiology
of the Heart

1.1 Definition

The heart is the pump in the cardiovascular system that forces blood through arteries, arterioles, capillaries, and veins, ensuring adequate circulation to tissues and organs throughout the body. Oxygenated blood moves away from the heart through the arterial system supplying oxygen and nutrients to cells (Figure 1.1). Through capillary action, gas and nutrients are exchanged for waste from cells. Waste is distributed through the venial system to organs that extract waste from blood where waste is excreted from the body. Deoxygenated blood returns to the heart, where it is pumped to the lungs for reoxygenation.

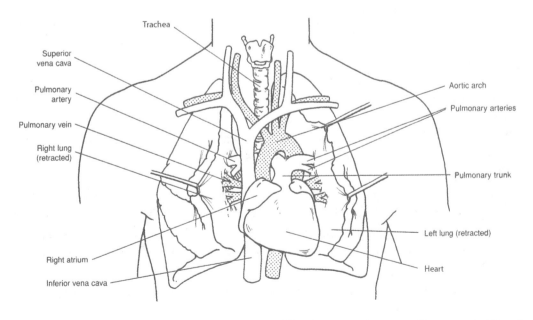

Figure 1.1 The heart pumps blood into arteries supplying tissues and organs with oxygenated blood.

1.2   Anatomy of the Heart

The heart is positioned in the middle of the chest cavity, called the *mediastinum,* on a tilt where the narrow portion of the heart, called the *apex,* is downward toward the left hip. The broader end of the heart, called the *base,* is toward the right shoulder. The terms used to describe anatomical positions are:

- **Anterior:** Front, posterior to the sternum
- **Posterior:** Back, anterior to the spine
- **Lateral:** Along the mid-axillary line
- **Inferior:** Superior to the diaphragm

Position of the Heart

The heart is the size of a fist, weighing approximately 310 g for males and 250 g for females. On average, the heart weighs 11 oz. The heart is slightly rotated to the left within the thoracic cavity, causing the right side of the heart to be more anterior (front, posterior to the sternum). Two-thirds of the heart lies on the left side and the remaining third on the right side.

- The base (top) of the heart is positioned beneath the second intercostal space (ICS).
- The apex (bottom pointed end) of the heart is located beneath the fifth ICS along the mid-clavicular line.
- The point of maximum impulse (PMI) is a ventricular contraction (heartbeat or systole) and is detected at the apex of the heart. This is the point where the apex beat can be felt. It is the product of the heart moving forward and striking the chest wall during systole.
- PMI can be displaced downward and laterally (along the mid-axillary line) if the patient has left ventricular hypertrophy (LVH) (thickening of the myocardium of the left ventricle) or cardiac tamponade (fluid collecting in the pericardial space).

Heart Chambers

The heart has four chambers:

1. **Right Atrium:** Positioned in the upper right side of the heart, the right atrium is a temporary storage chamber for returned venous blood. This ensures that blood is available for the right ventricle.
2. **Right Ventricle:** Positioned in the lower right side of the heart, the right ventricle is the pumping chamber for pulmonary circulation containing deoxygenated (70% saturated) blood.
3. **Left Atrium:** Positioned in the upper left side of the heart, the left atrium is a temporary storage chamber for oxygenated blood (100% saturated). This ensures that oxygenated blood is available for the left ventricle.
4. **Left Ventricle:** Positioned in the lower left side of the heart, the left ventricle is the pumping chamber for systemic circulation.

Pericardium

The heart is contained in a two-layer sac called the *pericardium*.

- The outer layer contains fibrous tissue that anchors the pericardium and heart to surrounding structures.

- The inner layer is divided into two layers called the *outer parietal layer* and *inner visceral layer*. Between these layers is fluid that provides a slippery surface for cardiac contractions (Figure 1.2).

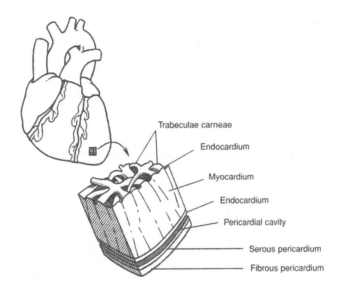

Trabeculae carneae
Endocardium
Myocardium
Endocardium
Pericardial cavity
Serous pericardium
Fibrous pericardium

Figure 1.2 The heart structure includes the pericardium, epicardium, myocardium, and endocardium.

Heart Wall

The wall of the heart is composed of three layers (see Figure 1.2).

1. **Epicardium:** This is the outermost layer and is the visceral layer of the serous pericardium.
2. **Myocardium:** This is the middle muscular layer that consists of cardiac muscles that contract and Purkinje fibers that conduct nerve impulses to cardiac muscle.
3. **Endocardium:** This is the thin, smooth lining of the heart that is continuous with the lining of blood vessels. Disruption of the endocardium by an infection (endocarditis) or congenital defect increases the risk for embolic stroke.

1.3   Heart Valves

Blood flows into the heart through valves. There are four valves (Figure 1.3).

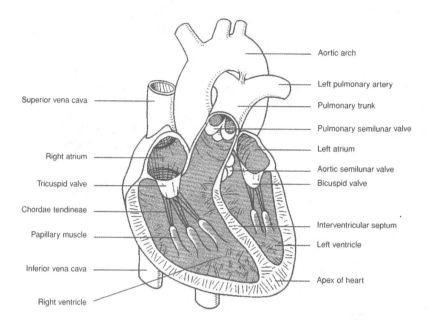

Figure 1.3 The flow of blood through the heart is controlled by four valves.

Tricuspid Valve (atrioventricular valve, AV)

The Tricuspid valve consists of three cusps that deliver blood from the right atrium to the right ventricle. The cusps prevent blood from backflowing into the right atrium.

- **Tricuspid Stenosis:** Narrowing of the tricuspid valve, usually as a result of rheumatic heart disease, causing increased pressure in the right atrium, resulting in thickening of the right atrium muscle or dilation of the right atrium. Systemic congestion or dependent edema might also result.

- **Tricuspid Regurgitation (TR):** An incompetent tricuspid valve results in a backflow of blood, called a *retrograde flow,* from the right ventricle into the right atrium. This condition is common in the late stages of right heart failure and also may be caused by inferior wall myocardial infarction involving the right ventricle. Tricuspid regurgitation might be the result of a transmural infarct, which is an infarct involving full thickness of the right ventricle, through to the papillary muscle in the myocardium.

Pulmonary Valve (semilunar valve)

The pulmonary valve facilitates blood flow between the right ventricle and pulmonary artery. This valve prevents backflow of blood from the pulmonary artery into the right ventricle.

Pulmonary valve stenosis-narrowing can occur around the valve during fetal development or later in life, usually as a result of rheumatic fever.

Pulmonary regurgitation is an incompetent pulmonic valve that allows blood to flow back into the right ventricle. The right ventricle is a low-pressure chamber. Increased pressure in the right chamber that results in increased volume causes right ventricular failure and leads to dependent edema, jugular venous distention, ascites, and hepatomegaly. These conditions can also occur as a result of pulmonary hypertension or endocarditis.

Mitral Valve (bicuspid valve)

The mitral valve uses two cusps to control blood flow between the left atrium and left ventricle. The cusps prevent a backflow of blood from the left ventricle to the left atrium.

- **Mitral Valve Regurgitation (MVR):** This is blood flowing back (retrograde) from the left ventricle to the left atrium, resulting in acute pulmonary edema. MVR is caused by:
  - Chronic rheumatoid heart disease
  - Mitral valve prolapse
  - Ischemic heart disease
  - Calcification of the mitral annulus
  - Infective endocarditis
  - Left ventricular dilation
    - *Left ventricular dilation* increases regurgitation of blood into the left atrium, causing enlargement of the left atrium and atrial dysrhythmias commonly seen with atrial enlargement.
- **Mitral Stenosis:** Narrowing of the mitral valve opening to 1.1 to 1.7 cm^2 as a result of rheumatic heart disease. This condition is asymptomatic until the later stage when atrial fibrillation signals that something is wrong.

Aortic Valve

The aortic valve controls blood flow between the left ventricle and the aorta and prevents blood from flowing back from the aorta into the left ventricle. The aortic valve has three leaflets.

Aortic Stenosis (AS)

This is the narrowing of the aortic valve caused by wear and tear and scarring from infections, and may be congenital. Aortic stenosis results in an increase in the pressure needed to move blood forward. This increase in pressure causes the left ventricle to become hypertrophied, predisposing the patient to left ventricular failure. Stenosis is not significant until the valve opening is reduced by 50%. The most common symptoms of aortic valve stenosis are chest pain, dyspnea, and syncope.

Aortic Incompetence

This occurs when a defect in the aortic valve permits regurgitation of blood from the aorta into the left ventricle. Aortic incompetence is caused by congenital defects, aging, aortic dissection, and infective endocarditis. The patient experiences chest pain with exertion, syncope, and difficulty breathing. The patient does not become symptomatic until the regurgitation is significant.

Bicuspid Aortic Valve (BAV)

Patients with this abnormal finding should be referred for ascending aortic aneurysm screening, due to the genetic link between having a BAV and an ascending aortic aneurysm. The aneurysm may not need surgical intervention, but monitoring the aneurysm can prevent a future dissection and rupture.

Papillary Muscles and Chordae

Chordae (see Figure 1.3) are tendons that connect the papillary muscles to the tricuspid valve and the mitral valve to the ventricular wall and floor. These are sometimes referred to as *heart strings*. Chordae break or papillary muscle rupture are conditions that can cause malfunction of the tricuspid and mitral valve, causing a backflow of blood and resulting in pulmonary edema, systemic congestion, cardiogenic shock, and interstitial edema.

1.4   Physiology of the Heart

Cardiac muscle fibers in the myocardium are connected by an intercalated disc at the site where plasma membranes intermesh. This enables cardiac muscle fibers to function as a single unit when contracting the heart. However, the atria are electrically insulated from the ventricles (Figure 1.4).

- **Sinoatrial (SA) Node:** Located in the upper right wall of the right atrium, the SA node generates an action potential that initiates the cardiac cycle.

- **Atrioventricular (AV) Node:** Located in the lower interatrial septum, the AV node causes a slight delay in the action potential before passing the action potential to the ventricles.

- **Bundle of His (AV bundle):** The bundle of His receives the action potential from the AV node and transmits the action to the ventricles through the left and right bundle branches.

- **Purkinje Fibers:** These are fibers with a large diameter that conduct the action potential from the interventricular septum through the apex to the ventricles.

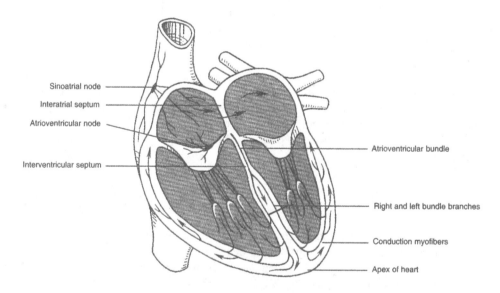

Figure 1.4 Contraction of cardiac muscle is controlled by the cardiac conduction system.

The Working Chambers

The heart pumps blood through four chambers, ensuring that deoxygenated blood flows to the lungs for gas exchange and to systemic tissues for nourishment and oxygenation (Figure 1.5).

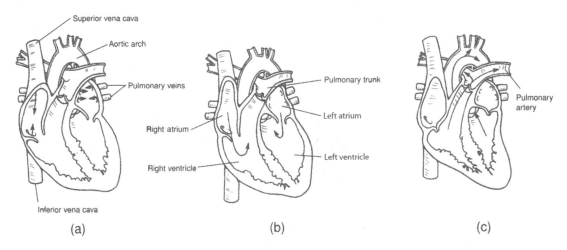

Figure 1.5 Blood flows through the heart, forcing deoxygenated blood to the lungs and oxygenated blood to the system.

- **Right Atrium:** Receives mixed venous blood (70% saturated with O_2) from the superior vena cava, inferior vena cava, and the coronary sinus.

- **Tricuspid Valve (right AV valve):** Separates the right atrium from the right ventricle. Mixed venous blood from the right atrium flows through the tricuspid value into the right ventricle.

- **Right Ventricle:** Pressure from the mixed venous blood in the right ventricle forces the tricuspid valve closed, preventing backflow of blood into the right atrium. Mixed venous blood leaves the right ventricle through the pulmonic valve into the pulmonary artery when the right ventricle contracts. The pulmonary artery delivers mixed venous blood to the lungs, where gas is exchanged.

  ○ Failure of the right ventricle results in interstitial edema or dependent edema.

- **Left Atrium:** Oxygenated blood is delivered by the pulmonary vein into the left atrium.

  ○ 70% to 80% of oxygenated blood passively fills the left ventricle because of increased pressure in the left atria as blood returns from the vena cava and pulmonary vein.

  ○ The atrium contracts, delivering the remaining 20% to 30% of oxygenated blood into the ventricles. This is referred to as the *atrial kick*. The atrial kick is lost in rhythms in which there is no atrial contraction. These patients can be symptomatic when going into an atrial dysrhythmia such as afibrillation, especially if they have a low ejection fraction, $<30\%$.

- **Left Ventricle:** Oxygenated blood flows from the left atrium through the mitral valve into the left ventricle. Pressure from oxygenated blood in the left ventricle causes the mitral valve to close, preventing backflow of blood into the left atrium. Oxygenated blood leaves the left ventricle through the aortic valve and flows into the aorta when the left ventricle contracts, causing oxygenated blood to enter the systematic circulation system.

  ○ Failure of the left ventricle results in fluid backup into the pulmonary system, resulting in congestive heart failure and, if severe enough, pulmonary edema.

1.5   Coronary Circulation

Coronary circulation supplies blood to cardiac tissue through the right and left coronary arteries from the aortic root in the ascending aorta located near the aortic valve (Figure 1.6). The number of vessels in coronary

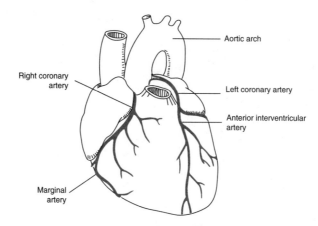

Figure 1.6 Blood is supplied to the heart through the coronary circulation system.

circulation and the location of these vessels varies depending on the patient. Disease of coronary circulation can quickly lead to myocardial infarction (heart attack).

Coronary Arteries

- **Epicardial coronary arteries:** The right and left coronary arteries branch into the epicardial coronary arteries on the epicardial surface (Figure 1.7).
  - ○ Epicardial coronary arteries autoregulate by dilating and constricting to meet the demands of the cardiac muscle.
  - ○ Atherosclerosis (narrowing of the artery) occurs when autoregulation fails, leading to angina.
- **Subendocardial coronary arteries:** The epicardial coronary arteries penetrate the myocardium and branch into the subendocardial coronary arteries (Figure 1.8).
  - ○ Subendocardial coronary arteries compress during systole and open during diastoles, enabling the arteries to fill with blood.

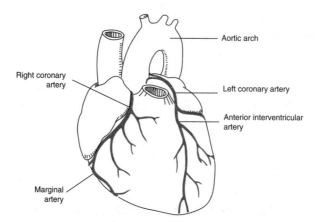

Figure 1.7 The epicardial coronary arteries receive blood from the left and right coronary arteries.

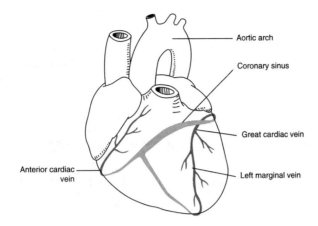

Figure 1.8 The subendocardial coronary arteries provide blood to the myocardium.

- **Right Coronary Artery (RCA):** This branches into the right marginal artery and the posterior descending artery (in 90% of the population). The right coronary artery supplies blood to the following:
  - Posterior wall of the left ventricle
  - Right atrium
  - Right ventricles
  - Inferior wall of the left ventricles
  - One-third of the posterior interventricular septum
  - SA node (in 55% of the population)
  - AV node (bundle of His—90% of the population)
- **Left Coronary Artery (LCA):** The left coronary artery branches into the left main coronary artery, which has the diameter of a drinking straw. The left main coronary artery branches into the following:
  - *Left Anterior Descending Artery:* This supplies blood to:
    - The anterolateral wall of the left ventricle
    - Two-thirds of the anterior interventricular septum
    - The right bundle branch
    - The anterior fascicles of the left bundle branch
  - *Left Circumflex Artery:* This supplies blood to:
    - The left atrium
    - The anterolateral wall of the left ventricle
  - *Posterior Descending Artery:* This supplies blood to:
    - The posterior wall of the left ventricle (in 10% of the population)

Collateral Circulation

Collateral circulation consists of blood vessels aside from coronary arteries whose purpose is to dilate when blockage affects the main coronary artery circulated, thereby providing a route to bypass the blockage. Collateral circulation may or may not be adequate to provide sufficient oxygenated blood to cardiac tissue.

Cardiac Veins

Cardiac veins run parallel to coronary arteries and remove deoxygenated blood from cardiac tissue. Deoxygenated blood carried by cardiac veins drain into the coronary sinus and then into the right atrium. Some deoxygenated blood flows from the cardiac veins directly into the right atrium.

1.6 Cardiac Innervation (the nerves that control the heart)

The heart is stimulated by the autonomic nervous system (Figure 1.9), which regulates involuntary muscle contraction.

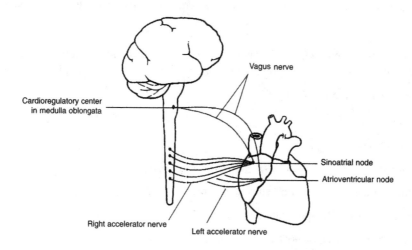

Figure 1.9 The autonomic nervous system stimulates the heart to contract.

Sympathetic Nervous System

The sympathetic nervous system accelerates cardiac contractions in response to the body's need for an increase in oxygenated blood.

- Efferent nerves innervate (supply an organ with nerves) the atrium and the SA node.

- When the catecholamine norepinephrine (a neurotransmitter) is released, the efferent nerves are stimulated, causing increased cardiac contractions. This is called *positive inotropy*.

- Increased amounts of catecholamine norepinephrine result in an increased velocity of AV nodal conduction. This is called *positive dromotrophy*.

- Increased velocity of conduction increases heart rate. This is called a *positive chronotrope*.

Parasympathetic Nervous System

The parasympathetic nervous system decelerates cardiac contractions in response to the body's need for a decrease in oxygenated blood.

- The right vagal nerve (CNX) innervates the SA node.
- The left vagal nerve innervates the AV node.

Acetylcholine is released when the body no longer requires a high level of oxygenated blood for tissues. When acetylcholine is released, the right and left vagal nerves are stimulated, resulting in a decrease in the velocity of conduction of cardiac muscle and therefore a decrease in heart rate.

1.7　Chest Pain

The sensation of chest pain that is related to the heart is called *angina pain,* which is transmitted by sensor nerve fibers located in T1 through T4 of the spine.

Cardiac Pain

Cardiac pain tends to be referred to areas shared by the same sensory nerves found in T1 through T4, dermatomes (Figure 1.10). The dermatome is an area of skin supplied by the same single spinal nerve. This shared area where referred pain is realized includes:

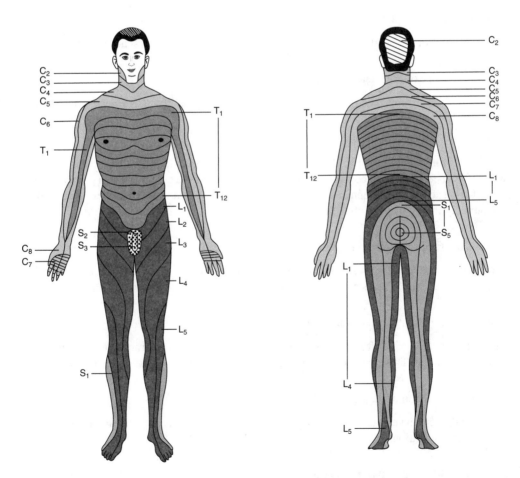

Figure 1.10 The dermatome is an area of skin that is shared by a single spinal nerve and is where referred pain is realized.

- Chest wall

- Epigastric

- Sternum

- Jaw

- Scapula

- Arm

- Hands

- Wrists

Solved Problems

Anatomy of the Heart

1.1 What is the narrow portion of the heart called?

The narrow portion of the heart is called the apex.

1.2 Where is the base of the heart positioned?

The base (top) of the heart is positioned beneath the second intercostal space (ICS).

1.3 Where is the apex of the heart positioned?

The apex (bottom pointed end) of the heart is located beneath the fifth ICS along the mid-clavicular line.

1.4 Where is the point of maximum impulse?

The point of maximum impulse (PMI) is the ventricular contraction (heartbeat), and is detected at the apex of the heart. PMI can be displaced down and lateral (along the mid-axillary line) if the patient has left ventricular hypertrophy (LVH) (thickening of the myocardium of the left ventricle) or cardiac tamponade (fluid collecting in the pericardial space).

1.5 What is the function of the right atrium?

Positioned in the upper right side of the heart, the right atrium is a temporary storage chamber for deoxygenated blood. This ensures that blood is available for the right ventricle.

1.6 What is the function of the left atrium?

Positioned in the upper left side of the heart, the left atrium is a temporary storage chamber for oxygenated blood. This ensures that oxygenated blood is available for the left ventricle.

1.7 What is the function of the right ventricle?

Positioned in the lower right side of the heart, the right ventricle is the pumping chamber for pulmonary circulation, containing deoxygenated blood.

1.8 What is the function of the left ventricle?

Positioned in the lower left side of the heart, the left ventricle is the pumping chamber for systemic circulation.

1.9   What is the myocardium?

The myocardium is the middle muscular layer that consists of cardiac muscle that contracts and Purkinje fibers that conduct nerve impulses to cardiac muscle.

Heart Valves

1.10   What is tricuspid stenosis?

Tricuspid stenosis is the narrowing of the tricuspid valve, usually as a result of rheumatic heart disease and causing increased pressure in the right atrium. This results in thickening of the right atrium muscle or dilation of the right atrium. Systemic congestion or dependent edema might also occur.

1.11   What is mitral valve regurgitation?

Mitral valve regurgitation (MVR) is blood flowing back (retrograde) from the left ventricle to the left atrium, resulting in acute pulmonary edema.

1.12   What might cause MVR?

Some causes of MVR are chronic rheumatoid heart disease, mitral valve prolapse, ischemic heart disease, calcification of the mitral annulus, infective endocarditis, and left ventricular dilation.

1.13   What is the function of chordae?

Chordae are tendons that connect the papillary muscles to the tricuspid valve and the mitral valve to the ventricular wall and floor.

Physiology of the Heart

1.14   What is the function of the SA node?

The sinoatrial (SA) node generates an action potential that initiates the cardiac cycle.

1.15   What is the function of the AV node?

The atrioventricular (AV) node causes a slight delay in the action potential before passing the action potential to the ventricles.

1.16   What is the function of the bundle of His?

The bundle of His receives the action potential from the AV node and transmits the action to the ventricles through the left and right bundle branches.

1.17   How does the right ventricle function?

Pressure of deoxygenated blood in the right ventricle forces the tricuspid valve to close, preventing backflow of blood into the right atrium. Deoxygenated blood leaves the right ventricle through the pulmonic valve and flows into the pulmonary artery when the right ventricle contracts. The pulmonary artery delivers deoxygenated blood to the lungs where gas is exchanged.

1.18   What is the atrial kick?

The atrium contracts, delivering the remaining 20% to 30% of oxygenated blood into the ventricles. This is referred to as the atrial kick. The atrial kick is lost in rhythms where there is no atrial contraction. These patients are symptomatic when going into an atrial dysrhythmia such as afibrillation.

1.19   What might occur if the right ventricle fails?

Failure of the right ventricle results in interstitial edema or dependent edema.

Coronary Circulation

1.20   What is the function of epicardial coronary arteries?

The right and left coronary arteries branch into the epicardial coronary arteries on the epicardial surface. Epicardial coronary arteries autoregulate by dilating and constricting to meet the demands of the cardiac muscle.

1.21   What is supplied blood by the right coronary artery?

The right coronary artery supplies blood to the posterior wall of the left ventricle, right atrium, right ventricle, inferior wall of the left ventricle, one-third of the posterior interventricular septum, SA node (55% of the population), and AV node (bundle of His—90% of the population).

1.22   What is supplied by the left circumflex artery?

The left circumflex artery supplies blood to the left atrium and the anterolateral wall of the left ventricle.

1.23   What is the function of collateral circulation?

Collateral circulation consists of blood vessels aside from coronary arteries whose purpose is to dilate when blockage affects the main coronary artery circulated, thereby providing a route to bypass the blockage.

1.24   Where do cardiac veins terminate?

Deoxygenated blood carried by cardiac veins drains into the coronary sinus and then into the right atrium. Some deoxygenated blood flows from the cardiac veins directly into the right atrium

1.25   Where do the efferent nerves innervate in the heart?

Efferent nerves innervate the atrium and SA node.

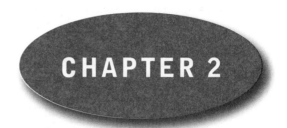

CHAPTER 2

Electrophysiology

2.1 Definition

Electrophysiology is the study of the electrical properties of tissues and cells. The electrical properties of cardiac muscle cause cardiac muscles to depolarize (contract) and repolarize (relax), resulting in a pumping action that forces blood throughout the body. An electrocardiograph (ECG) is a recording device that measures the electrophysiologic activity of the heart.

2.2 Cardiac Cells

The heart is composed of striated involuntary muscles called cardiac muscles. Cells in cardiac muscles are referred to as cardiomyocytes and are also known as pacemaker cells. Cardiomyocytes have three properties:

1. **Automaticity:** Cardiomyocytes are able to initiate an electrical impulse without influence directly from the nervous system.

2. **Excitability:** Cardiomyocytes respond to electrical impulses initiated by the nervous system such as to increase or decrease contractions depending on the body's requirements.

3. **Conductivity:** Cardiomyocytes transmit impulses to other cardiomyocytes, resulting in a coordinated depolarization and repolarization among cardiomyocytes.

Depolarization and Repolarization

Depolarization causes cardiac muscles to contract and repolarization causes cardiac muscles to return to their original position. Depolarization and repolarization are caused by movement of electrolytes into and out of cardiomyocytes (Figure 2.1).

- *Electrolytes:* An electrolyte is any substance containing free ions that make the substance conductive. Sodium and potassium are electrolytes used for electrical activity in cells.

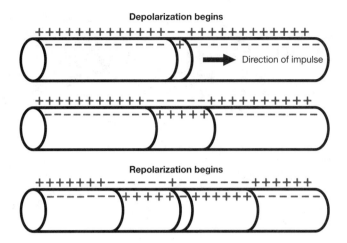

Figure 2.1 Cardiac muscle pumps blood by depolarization and repolarization.

- *Sodium-Potassium Pump:* The sodium-potassium pump traverses the cell membrane and uses adenosine-triphosphatase (ATP), an enzyme that uses metabolic energy to actively transport free ions into and out of the cell, thereby controlling electrical activity of the cell.

- *Depolarization:* Potassium (K), which is normally found inside a cell in higher concentrations than the blood, is moved out of the cell and replaced with sodium (Na), which is normally in lower concentrations in the cell. Sodium is normally found outside a cell. This exchange of electrolytes causes cardiomyocytes cardiac muscle to depolarize (contract).

- *Repolarization:* Cardiac muscle is depolarized. Sodium is inside the cell and potassium is outside the cell. Repolarization occurs when potassium returns inside the cell and sodium moves outside the cell, resulting in the cardiac muscle returning to a resting state.

Electrolyte Levels and Depolarization/Repolarization

Depolarization and repolarization may be altered by abnormal levels of electrolytes in the body, which can affect the conduction of impulses. These electrolytes are:

- **Sodium:** Sodium is the primary cation, a positively charged ion, located in the extracellular space, and is responsible for regulation of blood and body fluids, transmission of nerve impulses, and cardiac activity. Abnormal levels can have a profound effect on neurologic status. Normal levels are 135 mEq/L to 145 mEq/L.

  - *Hyponatremia:* A serum sodium level of <135 mEq/L

    - The underlying cause of hyponatremia is assessed by measuring the serum and urine osmolality. Osmolality is the concentration of the fluid. The higher the osmolality, the more concentrated the fluid is; the lower the osmolality, the more diluted it is.

    - Serum Osmolality: This is used to differentiate among hyponatremia, pseudohyponatremia, and hypertonic.

    - Urine Osmolality: This is used to differentiate between primary polydipsia and impaired free water excretion. Polydipsia is excessive thirst, resulting in excessive drinking.

      - Urine osmolality >20 mmol/L and the patient is dehydrated.

- Addison disease

- Excess diuresing or water excretion by the kidneys

- Renal failure

♦ Urine osmolality >500 mmol/L and the patient is not edematous or dehydrated.

- Syndrome of inappropriate antidiuretic hormone (SIADH)

- Water intoxication—Drinking too much water, resulting in low sodium, nausea, vomiting, and cerebral edema

- Severe hypothyroidism—Disturbance with the thyroid, pituitary, or hypothalamus that results in low levels of the T4 hormone

- Glucocorticoid insufficiency—Insufficient amount of the body's naturally occurring steroids that are responsible for controlling inflammation

- Urine sodium concentration: This is used to differentiate among hypovolemia, hyponatremia, and SIADH.

♦ Urine sodium <20 mmol/L and the patient is dehydrated.

- Loss through diarrhea, vomiting, burns, trauma, or small bowel obstruction

- Nephrotic syndrome

- Cirrhosis

- Renal failure

- **Potassium:** Very low or very high levels of potassium can result in a life-threatening situation.

  ○ *Hypokalemia:* Serum potassium level <3.5 mEq/L

  - Hypokalemia amplifies other medical conditions on the ECG such as digitalis-induced arrhythmias, myocardial infarction (MI), or hypomagnesemia.

  - Hypokalemia does not cause arrhythmias.

  - ECG:

    ♦ T Wave: Flatten and/or inverse

    ♦ QT Wave: Prolonged

    ♦ U Wave: Prominent

  ○ *Hyperkalemia:* Serum potassium level >5.5 mEq/L

  - Hyperkalemia: Hyperkalemia is life threatening because it decreases cardiac conduction

  - ECG:

    ♦ May see changes when serum potassium level reaches 6.6 mEq/L

    ♦ Always see changes when serum potassium level is >8.0 mEq/L

    ♦ T Wave: Begins with peaked in V_2 and V_3 leads

    ♦ P Wave: Amplitude is lost

    ♦ PR Interval: Prolonged. Increased interval indicates cardiac conduction is slowing, leading to a complete heart block: >0.20 in a first-degree heart block.

- **Magnesium:** This is an electrolyte that is required for the operation of the sodium-potassium pump. Magnesium is also an intrinsic calcium blocker.

  ○ *Hypomagnesemia:* Serum magnesium level <1.4 mEq/L

    ▪ Causes early depolarization resulting in tachyarrhythmias, especially torsades de pointes (polymorphous ventricular tachycardia), which is life threatening, and QTI prolongation (Figure 2.2).

    ▪ Most commonly underdiagnosed electrolyte abnormality.

    ▪ A side effect of:

      ♦ Diuretic therapy

      ♦ Antibiotic therapy (decreased reabsorption of magnesium when aminoglycosides are administered to the patient)

      ♦ Diarrhea

  ○ *Hypermagnesemia:* Serum magnesium level >2.0 mEq/L

    ▪ High levels of magnesium decrease serum calcium.

    ▪ Hypermagnesemia is caused by:

      ♦ Renal impairment

      ♦ Adrenal insufficiency

      ♦ Hyperparathyroid

      ♦ Lithium intoxication

      ♦ Diabetic ketoacidosis (DKA)

    ▪ Hypermagnesemia can cause:

      ♦ Hyporeflexia (low reflexes) at serum levels >4 mEq/L

      ♦ First-degree AV block at serum levels >5 mEq/L (Figure 2.3)

      ♦ Complete heart block (CHB) at serum levels >10 mEq/L

      ♦ Cardiac arrest at serum levels >13 mEq/L

- **Calcium:** This is the most abundant electrolyte in the body and is involved in coagulation, neuromuscular transmission, and smooth muscle contraction. Ionized calcium is the biologically active form of calcium. Total serum calcium corrected to albumin levels is as useful as ionized calcium.

  ○ *Ionized Hypocalcemia:* The serum level of ionized calcium is <1.3 mmol/L. Ionized calcium is free calcium ions that are not bound to protein.

    ▪ Caused by:

      ♦ Depletion of magnesium

      ♦ Sepsis

      ♦ Alkalosis

      ♦ Transfusions

      ♦ Medication

        – Mithramycin (plicamycin), bisphosphonates, calcitonin, and oral or parental phosphate preparations and prolonged therapy with anticonvulsants such as diphenylhydantoin (phenytoin) or phenobarbital.

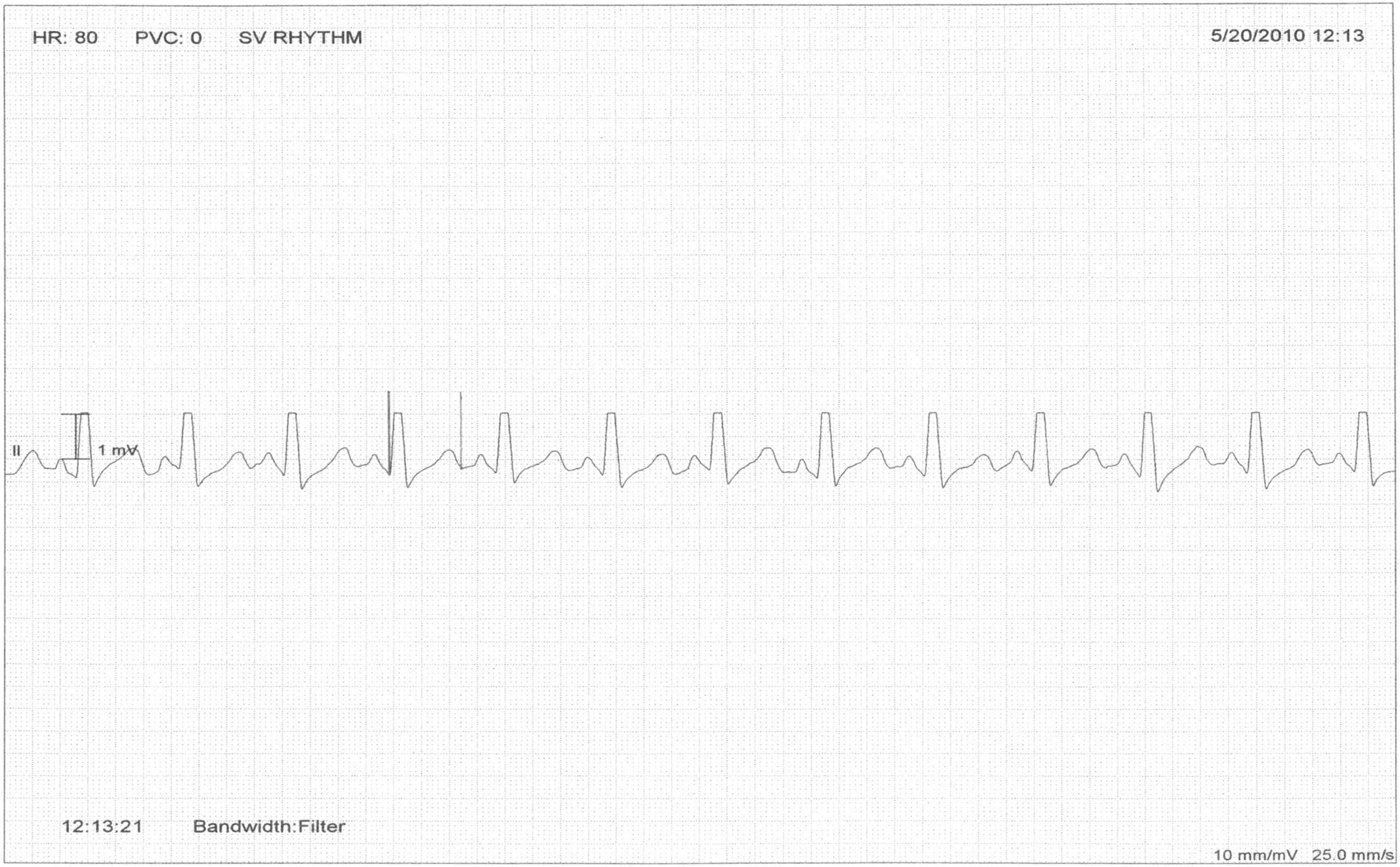

HR: 80   PVC: 0   SV RHYTHM   5/20/2010 12:13

II   1 mV

12:13:21   Bandwidth:Filter   10 mm/mV   25.0 mm/s

Figure 2.2 This strip shows a prolonged QT interval of 0.52 ms, indicating the most commonly underdiagnosed electrolyte abnormality.

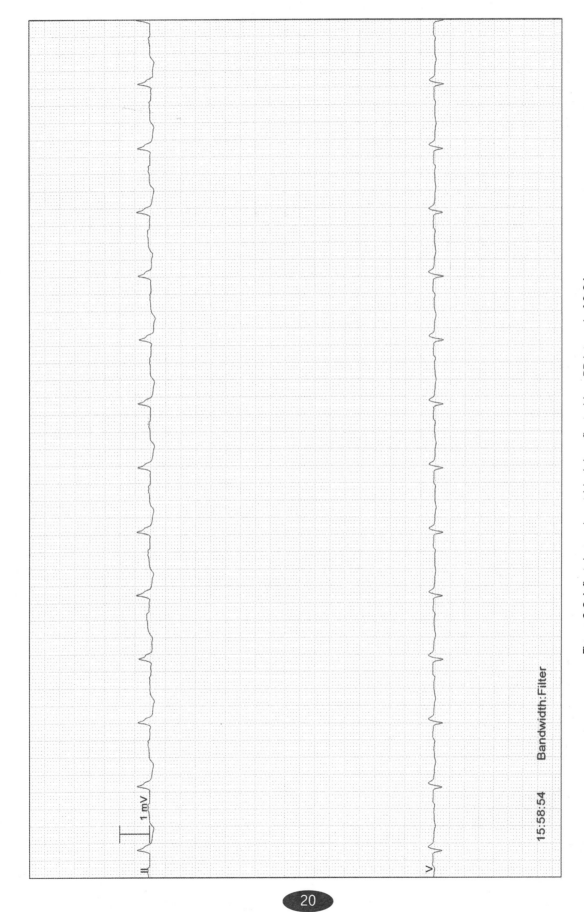

Figure 2.3 A first-degree heart block is reflected in a PR interval of 0.24 ms.

- ◆ Renal failure

- ◆ Pancreatitis

- ▪ Causes:

  - ◆ Hypotension

  - ◆ Decreased cardiac output

  - ◆ Ventricular ectopy (extra heartbeat originating in the lower chamber of the heart)

  - ◆ Heart blocks

- ▪ Cardiovascular affects:

  - ◆ Rarely seen in serum levels of 0.8 to 1.0 mmol/L

  - ◆ Typically seen in serum levels <0.65 mmol/L

- ○ *Ionized Hypercalcemia:* Serum level of ionized calcium is >2.5 mmol/L

  - ▪ Not as common as hypocalcemia

  - ▪ Severe hypercalcemia:

    - ◆ Total serum calcium: >14 mmol/L

    - ◆ Ionized serum calcium: >3.5 mmol/L

    - ◆ Caused by:

      - – Thyrotoxicosis (related to hyperthyroidism)

      - – Malignancy

      - – Medication

      - – Excessive vitamin D, alkaline antacids, diethylstilbestrol (DES), long-term use of diuretics, estrogens, and progesterone

      - – Cardiovascular affects:

        - - Hypovolemia—low circulating volume

        - - Hypotension—low blood pressure

      - – ECG:

        - - QT Interval: Shortened

2.3 Conduction System

The conduction system (Figure 2.4) of the heart transmits electrical impulses throughout the heart, causing depolarization and repolarization of cardiac muscle resulting in a pumping action that moves blood throughout the body. Table 2.1 contains the pathophysiologic changes that might occur during depolarization/repolarization and how these changes appear in an ECG strip.

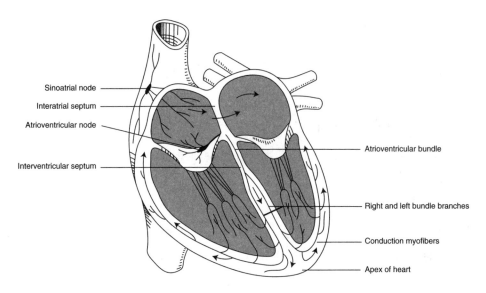

Figure 2.4 Transmission of electrical impulses throughout the heart is performed by the cardiac conduction system.

TABLE 2.1 Pathophysiologic Changes Seen in an ECG

Hypocalcemia	Prolonged QT interval
Hypercalcemia	Shortened QT interval
Hyperkalemia	Peaked T wave, PRI prolonged
Ischemia	T wave inversion
Transmural infarct	ST elevation
Subendocardial injury	ST depression
Acute pericarditis	Diffuse ST elevation

The Functioning Conduction System

- **SA Node:** The SA node, located in the upper right atrium, is the heart's intrinsic pacemaker generating impulses that cause depolarization at a rate between 60 and 100 impulses (beats) per minute.

- **Bachmann Bundles:** Impulse from the SA node is carried through interatrial pathways called the Bachmann bundles to the left atrium, resulting in the depolarization (contraction) of the left and right atria.

   - *ECG:* A P wave is generated.

   - *Internodal Pathways:* Internodal pathways carry the impulse through the right atrium to the AV node.

   - *AV Node:* The AV node is located in the right lower atrium at the interatrial septum and is the only communication pathway between the atria and the ventricles.

      - The AV node's intrinsic rate is 40 to 60 impulses per minute and is a backup source to generate the cardiac impulse if the SA node fails.

- The AV node slows the impulse to the ventricles allowing time for the atria to completely empty, which is referred to as the atrial kick.

- Atrial Fibrillation: Atrial fibrillation (afib) is the rapid depolarization and repolarization of the atrium. The AV node slows or blocks this impulse to the ventricles, reducing the likelihood of a rapid ventricle response (rapid heart rate).

- ECG: The PR interval represents the time it takes for the impulse to depolarize the atrium then travel to the AV node, where the impulse is detained briefly before being released to the bundle of His. The onset of atrial depolarization is the P wave, and the onset of ventricular depolarization is the Q wave.

- **Bundle of His:** The bundle of His carries the impulse to the left and right bundle branches, delivering the impulse to the Purkinje fibers.

- **Right Bundle Branches:** The right bundle branches carry the impulse to the right ventricle, causing the right ventricle to depolarize (contract).

- **Left Bundle Branches:** The left bundle branches carry the impulse to the left ventricle, causing the left ventricle to depolarize (contract).

- **ECG:** QRS wave complex, which is equal to the R wave, is produced.

- **Ventricular Repolarization:** Ventricular repolarization occurs at the end of ventricular depolarization.

  - *ECG:*

    - Beginning Ventricular Repolarization: An ST segment is produced.

    - Later Ventricular Repolarization: A T wave is produced.

    - Note: The U wave is produced following the T wave in 50% of patients.

- **Ventricular Depolarization/Repolarization:**

  - *ECG:* QT interval measures the duration between depolarization and repolarization of the ventricles.

2.4 Cardiac Cycle

The cardiac cycle consists of one sequence of depolarization and repolarization of the atria and ventricles. This is measured on an ECG by a P wave followed by a QRS complex and ending with a T wave, and is called the PQRST sequence (Figure 2.6).

- **Normal Sinus Rhythm (NSR):** Normal sinus rhythm is a series of the PQRST sequence.

- **R-R Interval:** Cardiac rhythm (heartbeat) is determined by measuring the R-R Interval, which is the distance between R waves on the ECG.

- **Isoelectric Line:** The isoelectric line, also known as a flat line, connects each PQRST sequence on an ECG. The isoelectric line represents the resting heart where no measurable electrical activity is occurring. Depolarization and repolarization are represented by elevations or depressions of the isoelectric line on the ECG.

- **Positive Deflection:** A positive deflection occurs when the line is elevated from the isoelectric line on the ECG. This represents measurable electrical activity of the heart.

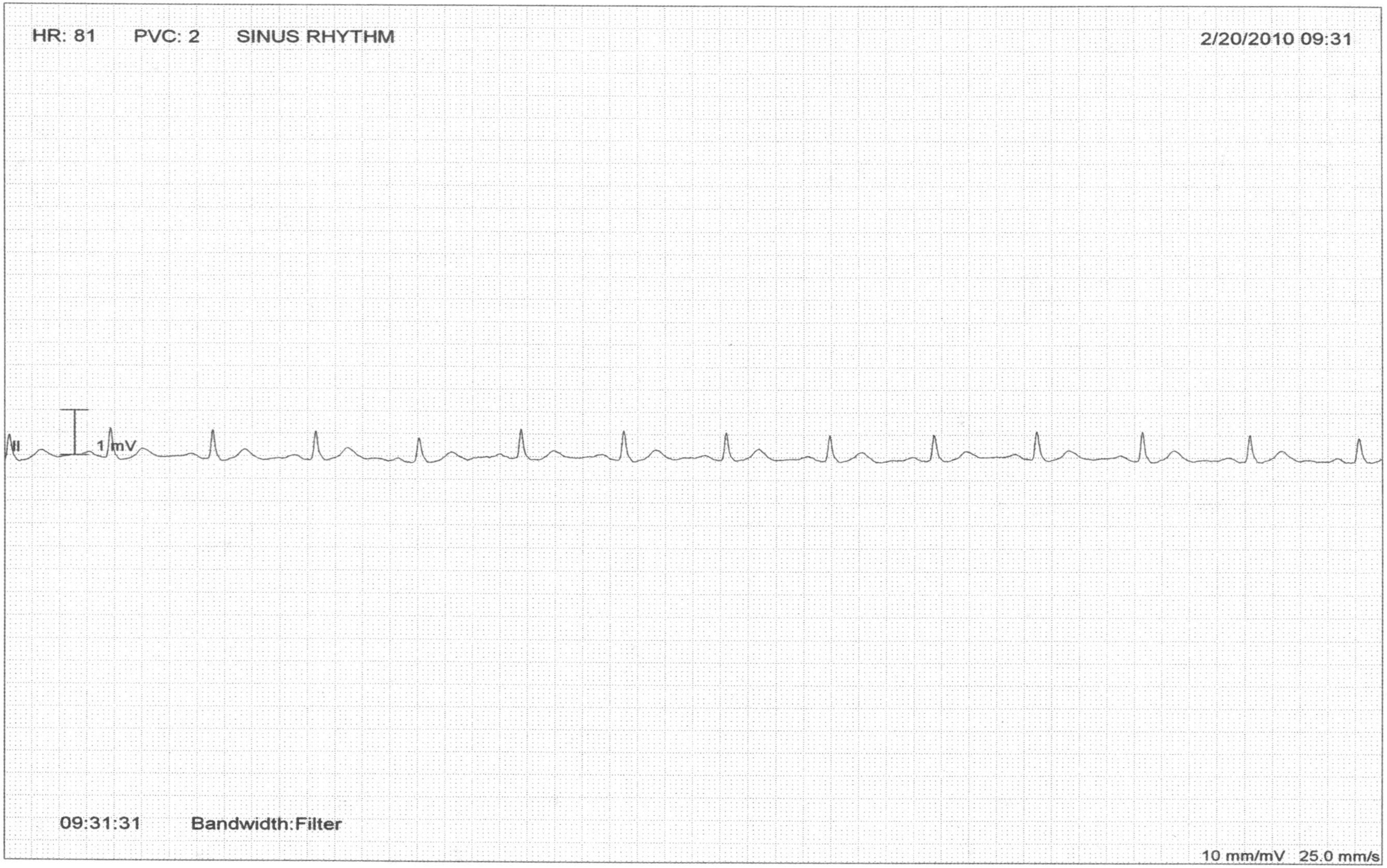

HR: 81   PVC: 2   SINUS RHYTHM

2/20/2010 09:31

1/mV

09:31:31   Bandwidth:Filter

10 mm/mV 25.0 mm/s

Figure 2.6 The normal sinus rhythm (NSR).

- **Negative Deflection:** Occurs when the line is depressed below the isoelectric line on the ECG. This represents measurable electrical activity of the heart.

The Refractory Period

The refractory period is the resting state of the heart when no measurable electrical activity occurs. This is the period when cardiac muscle prepares for the next impulse.

- **Threshold Potential:** Threshold potential is the moment when cardiac cells have sufficient electrical capability to depolarize.

- **Absolute Refractory Period:** Absolute refractory period occurs when cardiac cells are absolutely incapable of depolarization. Cells are still repolarizing and there is not enough threshold potential to depolarize the cells.

  - *ECG:* Absolute refractory period occurs during the QRS complex and carries through the middle of the T wave.

- **Relative Refractory Period:** Relative refractory period occurs when there is enough threshold potential for cardiac cells to depolarize.

  - *ECG:* Relative refractory period occurs at the second half of the T wave.

- **R-on-T Phenomenon:** The R-on-T phenomenon occurs when an impulse is generated during the T wave, which can result in the life-threatening condition of ventricular tachycardia. This happens as a result of a prolonged QT interval or a cardioversion (shocking the heart) not synchronized with the depolarization and repolarization of the heart.

- **Supernormal Period:** The supernormal period occurs immediately after the T wave. Weak stimulation during this period might cause an ectopic (extra) heartbeat, such as a premature atrial contraction or premature ventricular contraction.

Solved Problems

Cardiac Cells

2.1   What are cardiomyocytes?

Cardiomyocytes are cardiac cells, also known as pacemaker cells.

2.2   What is the automaticity of cardiac cells?

Automaticity occurs when cardiomyocytes are able to initiate an electrical impulse without direct influence from the nervous system.

2.3   What is the excitability of cardiomyocytes?

Excitability occurs when cardiomyocytes respond to electrical impulses initiated by the nervous system such as to increase or decrease contractions depending on the body's requirements.

2.4   What is the conductivity of cardiomyocytes?

Conductivity occurs when cardiomyocytes transmit impulses to other cardiomyocytes, resulting in a coordinated depolarization and repolarization among them.

2.5   What is depolarization?

Depolarization is the mechanism that causes cardiac muscles to contract.

2.6   What is repolarization?

Repolarization is the mechanism that results in cardiac muscles returning to their original position.

2.7   What causes depolarization and repolarization of cardiac muscles?

Depolarization and repolarization are caused by movement of electrolytes into and out of cardiomyocytes.

2.8   What are electrolytes?

Electrolytes are substances that contain free ions, making them conductive.

2.9   What electrolytes are used for electrical activity in cells?

Sodium and potassium are electrolytes used for electrical activity in cells.

2.10   What is the function of the sodium-potassium pump?

The sodium-potassium pump is an enzyme in the cell membrane that actively transports free ions into and out of the cell, thereby controlling the electrical activity of the cell.

2.11   What electrolyte action occurs during depolarization?

Potassium (K), which is normally found inside a cell, is moved out of the cell and replaced with sodium (Na). Sodium is normally found outside a cell. This exchange of electrolytes causes cardiomyocytes to depolarize (contract).

2.12   What electrolyte action occurs during repolarization?

Cardiac muscle is depolarized. Sodium is inside the cell and potassium is outside the cell. Repolarization occurs when potassium returns inside the cell and sodium moves outside the cell, resulting in the cardiac muscle returning to a resting state.

2.13   Does hypokalemia cause arrhythmias to be detected on an ECG?

No. Hypokalemia amplifies other medical conditions on the ECG such as digitalis-induced arrhythmias, myocardial infarction (MI), or hypomagnesemia.

2.14   Why is hyperkalemia life threatening?

Hyperkalemia is life threatening because it decreases cardiac conduction.

2.15   What is the function of magnesium?

Magnesium is an electrolyte that is required for the operation of the sodium-potassium pump.

2.16   What causes hypomagnesemia?

Hypomagnesemia is a side effect of diuretic therapy, antibiotic therapy (decreased reabsorption of magnesium when aminoglycosides are administered to the patient), and diarrhea.

2.17   What is ionized calcium?

Ionized calcium is the biologically active form of calcium.

Conduction System

2.18   What is the function of the conduction system?

The conduction system of the heart is responsible for transmitting electrical impulses throughout the heart to cause depolarization and repolarization of cardiac muscle, resulting in the pumping action that moves blood throughout the body.

2.19   What is the heart's intrinsic pacemaker?

The heart's intrinsic pacemaker is the SA node.

2.20   What is the function of the Bachman's bundle?

Impulses from the SA node are carried to the left atrium through an interatrial pathway called Bachmann's bundle, resulting in the depolarization (contraction) of the left and right atria.

2.21   What might occur if the AV node slows or is blocked?

Atrial fibrillation (afib) is the rapid depolarization and repolarization of the atrium. The AV node slows or blocks this impulse to the ventricles, reducing the likelihood of a rapid ventricular response.

2.22   What is an alternative function of the AV node?

The AV node is a backup source to generate the cardiac impulse if the SA node fails.

2.23   What is the function of the bundle of His?

The bundle of His carries the impulse to the left and right bundle branches, delivering the impulse to the Purkinje fibers.

The Cardiac Cycle

2.24   What is normal sinus rhythm?

Normal sinus rhythm is a series of the PQRST sequence, with appropriate timing and rest.

2.25   What is the isoelectric line on an ECG?

The isoelectric line, also known as a flat line, connects each PQRST sequence on an ECG. The isoelectric line represents the resting heart where no measurable electrical activity is occurring. Depolarization and repolarization are represented by elevations or depressions of the isoelectric line on the ECG.

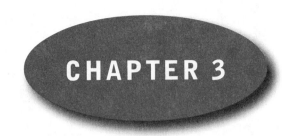

CHAPTER 3

Waveforms and Complexes

3.1 Definition

Electrical properties of cardiac muscle cause the pumping action by forcing blood throughout the body by depolarizing and repolarizing cardiac muscle. Normal cardiac action is recorded by the electrocardiograph (ECG) as a normal waveform. Atypical actions of the heart such as a defective heart valve or restricted cardiac circulation result in a change in the electrophysiology of the heart. This change is reflected in the waveforms recorded by the electrocardiograph.

3.2 Components of the ECG Tracing

The ECG tracing is an image of the electrophysiology of cardiac muscle in the form of a line that is automatically drawn on a graph paper by the electrocardiograph. Initially, the line is aligned to a baseline on the graph paper. This is referred to as zeroing or calibrating the ECG and is performed before recording a patient's ECG (Figure 3.1).

The baseline is called the isoelectric line, which is a straight horizontal line on the graph paper commonly called a flat line. The graph paper consists of small and large boxes. Each small box is 1 mm^2. There are five small boxes in one large box.

5 small= 1lg

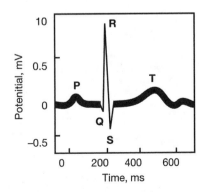

Figure 3.1 The ECG is calibrated before the patient's ECG is recorded.

When the electrophysiology of cardiac muscle is recorded, the electrocardiograph moves the graph paper at a rate of 12 mm/sec. This results in each small box passing the stylist every 40 ms and one large block every 200 ms.

Electrodes placed on the patient's body detect electrical changes in the electrophysiology of cardiac muscle. These electrical changes are transmitted through wires to the electrocardiograph and cause the ECG stylus to move vertically on the graph paper, drawing a line image that reflects the corresponding electrical changes in the electrophysiology of cardiac muscle. This image is recognized as the PQRST sequence that occurs over a measurable time frame.

3.3   P Wave

The P wave is the first deflection of the isoelectric line and starts when there is electrical activity at the SA node, signifying atrial depolarization. There is one P wave for every QRS complex; it appears upright and rounded (Figure 3.2).

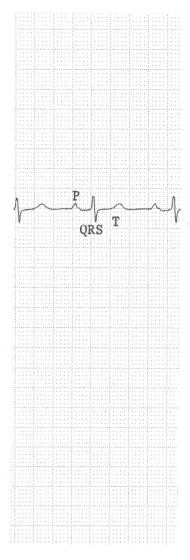

Figure 3.2 The P wave begins the deflection of the isoelectric line and is followed by the QRS complex and the T wave.

Normal P wave:

- Begins when the stylus leaves the isoelectric line and ends when the stylus returns to the isoelectric line

- Is no more than 2.5 mm in height (2.5 small boxes) because the atrium is a smaller muscle mass requiring less voltage to depolarize cells than with the ventricles

- Is no more than 0.10 seconds in width, less than three small boxes

- Measures the duration of atrial depolarization

Abnormal P wave caused by disrupted electrical conduction of the atrium:

- Multiple P waves for each QRS complex might indicate a second-degree heart block resulting in a blockage of the electrical signal.

- A tall, peaked P wave indicates right atrial enlargement (RAE), as seen in severe pulmonary disease such as chronic obstructive pulmonary disease, asthma, congenital heart disease, and acute pulmonary embolism.

- A wide and notched P wave indicates left atrial enlargement (LEA) as seen in left ventricular myopathies and mitral valve disease.

- An inverted or absent P wave indicates that the initial electrical impulse is originating other than by the SA node (ectopic in nature) and is seen in junctional rhythms.

3.4 PR Interval

The PR interval (PRI) (Figure 3.3) is the period between the end of the P wave and the beginning of the QRS complex. This is represented on the graph as the isoelectric line indicating the time the electrical impulse takes to travel to the ventricles after atrial repolarization.

- The normal PR interval is

  - Measured from the time the P wave returns to the isoelectric line to the start of the Q wave in the QRS complex

  - Between 0.12 seconds and 0.20 seconds, three to five small boxes

- The abnormal PR interval is

  - Shortened PRI (<0.12 seconds), indicating that:

    - A shorter path was taken to send the impulse to the ventricles.

    - An accessory pathway was used to send the impulse other than through the AV node, such as in Wolff-Parkinson-White disease.

    - The impulse begins from a site other than the SA node (ectopic site) that is closer than the SA node is to the AV node.

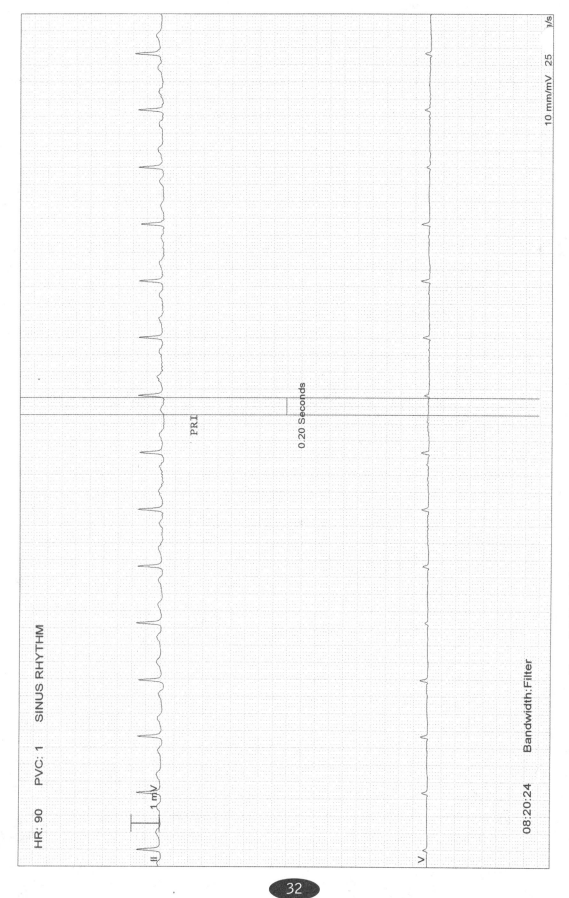

Figure 3.3 The PR interval measures the time the impulse takes to reach the ventricles.

- ○ Prolonged PRI (>0.20 seconds)

  - ▪ Slower conduction of the impulse through the AV node seen in:

    - ◆ Toxicity of medication that slows conduction (i.e., digitalis toxicity)

    - ◆ Aging

    - ◆ Hypothyroidism

    - ◆ Seen in a first-degree heart block rhythm

3.5   QRS Complex

The QRS complex (Figure 3.4) is a three-wave deflection of the isoelectric line that traces the electrical impulse after leaving the AV node and travels through the bundle of His resulting in ventricular depolarization. Ventricles are the largest muscles in the heart, requiring higher voltage than the atrials to depolarize, which is why the QRS complex is larger than the P wave.

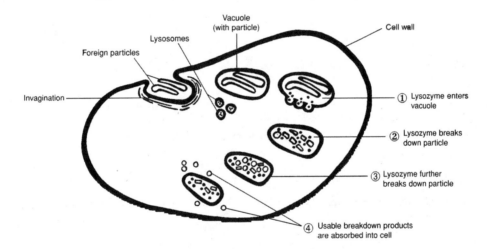

Figure 3.4 The QRS complex shows the impulse through the bundle of His.

- • The normal QRS complex is:

  - ○ Measured from the beginning of the Q wave to the end of the S wave when the S wave returns to the isoelectric line, which is called the J point.

  - ○ Difficult at times to locate the end of the S wave because of variations in the elevation/depression of the ST segment (see ST Segment).

  - ○ Identified by the width of the QRS line image on the graph. The isoelectric line is thicker (fatter) than the QRS line image on the graph.

  - ○ Predominantly positive in lead II

    - ▪ Duration is 0.04 to 0.10 seconds—one to two and a half small boxes.

    - ▪ The Q wave is a negative deflection (down).

    - ▪ The R wave is a positive deflection (up).

- The S wave is a negative deflection (down).

- The QRS complex is completely negative (down), which is call a QS complex.

  ○ Called an R Prime if the QRS complex has more than one R wave. This is written as R′

  ○ Called an S Prime if the QRS complex has more than one S wave. This is written as S′ (Figure 3.5)

  ○ Labeled as a separate wave, such as R′ and S′, if the QRS complex crosses the isoelectric line and if the QRS complex is not notched

  ○ Lowercase letters (s′ or r′) indicate an amplitude (height) <5 mm

  ○ Uppercase letters (S′ or R′) indicate an amplitude ≥5 mm

- The abnormal QRS complex is:

  ○ Notched QRS complex (Figure 3.6) indicates a bundle branch block where conduction through the bundle branches is blocked.

  ○ Widened QRS (>0.12 seconds) indicates early depolarization of the ventricles caused either by the impulse following an accessory pathway other than through the AV node or the initiating impulse is beginning in the ventricles (ectopic beat).

3.6 ST Segment

The ST segment is the time period between the end of ventricular depolarization and ventricular repolarization. The S wave returning to the isoelectric line represents the end of ventricular depolarization. The beginning of the T wave represents the beginning of ventricular repolarization.

- The normal ST segment is:

  ○ Measured from the beginning of the J point, which is the end of the QRS complex and the beginning of the T wave

    - Begin measuring one small box (0.04 seconds) past the J point.

- An abnormal ST segment (Figure 3.7) is characterized by:

  ○ An elevated ST segment:

    - Elevation >1 mm (one large square) in two or more leads has clinical significance.

    - Indicates a possible:

      ◆ Convex elevation indicates a myocardial infarction (MI).

      ◆ Concave elevation (>2 mm) indicates a nonacute MI relating to benign early ventricular repolarization or might indicate pericarditis.

      ◆ Horizontal elevation indicates MI.

      ◆ Distribution of ST elevations is related to ECG leads that are detecting the nonacute MI.

      ◆ Elevated ST segments in all leads indicate a cause other than MI such as pericarditis.

      ◆ Hyperkalemia and vasospasms (i.e., Prinzmetal's angina) also cause ST elevations.

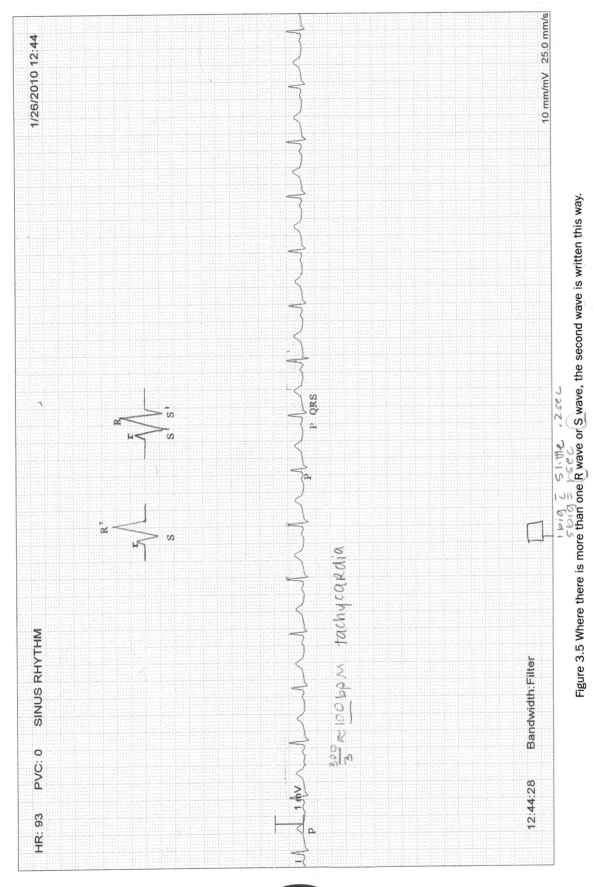

Figure 3.5 Where there is more than one R wave or S wave, the second wave is written this way.

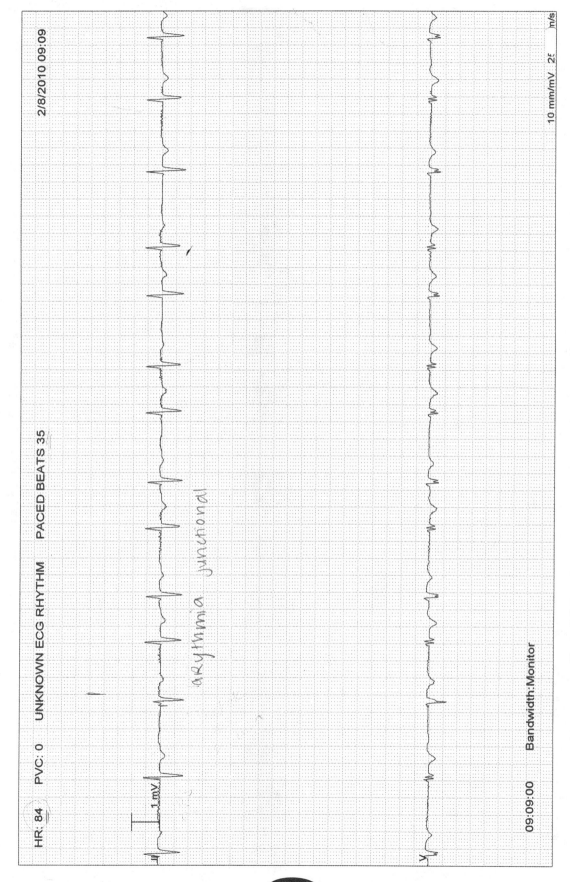

Figure 3.6 The notch in the QRS complex indicates a blockage of the bundle branch.

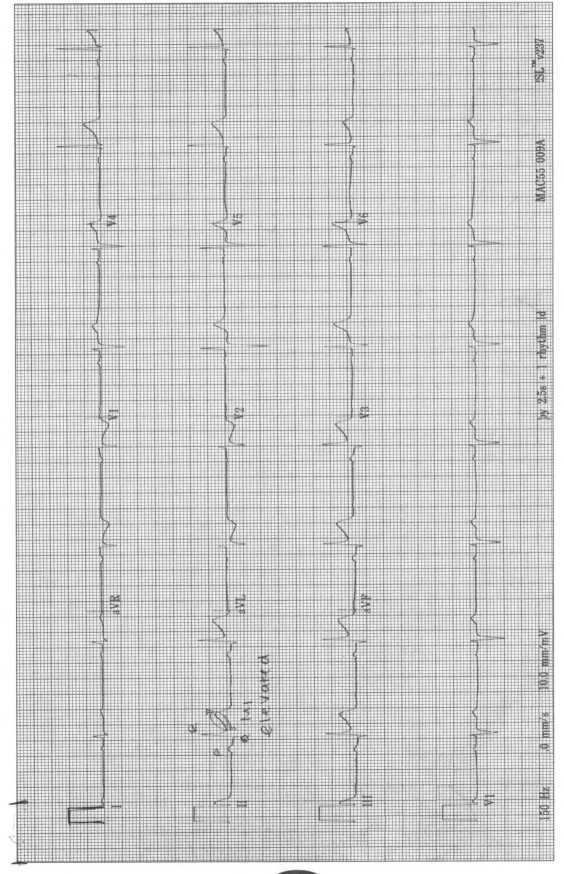

Figure 3.7 The ST wave is elevated in leads II, III, and AVF.

- o Depressed ST segment (Figure 3.8):

  - ▪ Can have a scooped-out appearance, a horizontal depression, or a down-sloping depression

  - ▪ Can be the result of reciprocal changes where corresponding leads have mirrored changes (one lead shows a depressed ST segment and another lead shows an elevated ST segment)

  - ▪ Indicates a possible:

    - ◆ Non-Q wave MI

    - ◆ Subendocardial MI

    - ◆ Ischemia (transient) resolved with rest, nitrates, morphine that encourages reperfusion

    - ◆ Hypokalemia (depression is <1 mm and has a normal T wave that is called a nonspecific ST abnormality)

    - ◆ Hypothermia (also lengthens the PR interval and the QT interval)

3.7 T Wave

The T wave begins at the end of the ST interval and has a gradual upward slope from the isoelectric line followed by a quick drop to the isoelectric line. The T wave represents the latter phase of ventricular repolarization.

- • A normal T wave has:

  - o An amplitude (height) of <5 mm.

- • An abnormal T wave:

  - o A generalized tall peaked T wave indicates hyperkalemia.

  - o A localized tall peaked T wave indicates MI.

  - o An inverted T wave indicates:

    - ▪ Evolving infarction

    - ▪ Chronic pericarditis

    - ▪ Conduction block

    - ▪ Ventricular hypertrophy

    - ▪ Acute cerebral disease

  - o A flattened T wave is nonspecific.

3.8 QT Interval

The QT interval (QTI) extends from the beginning of the QRS complex to the end of the T wave (Figure 3.9). This represents the complete cycle of ventricular depolarization/repolarization. The QT interval has an inverse relationship with the heart rate. As the heart rate increases, the QT interval decreases. As the heart rate decreases, the QT interval increases.

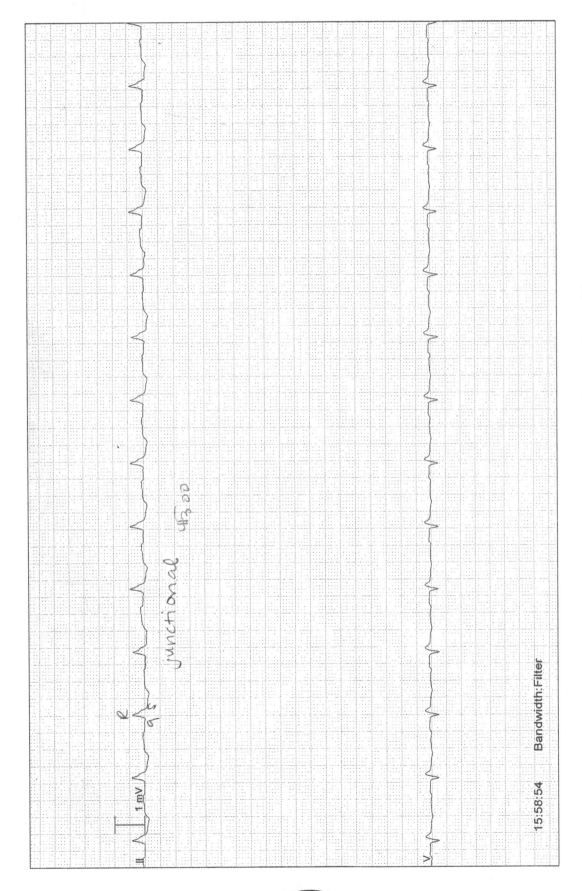

Figure 3.8 The ST segment is depressed when there is an inverted T wave.

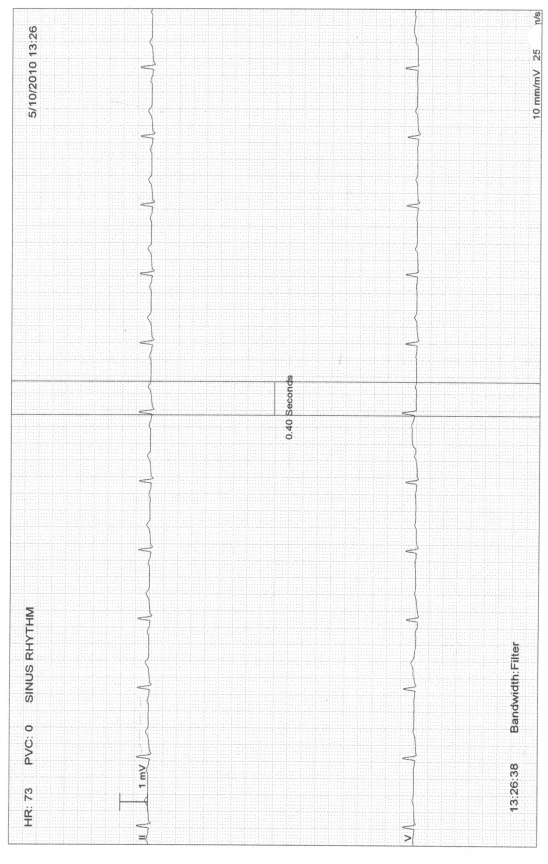

Figure 3.9 The QT interval increases as the heart rate decreases.

Correcting QT interval measurement:

1. Measure the QT interval by adjusting the QT interval to the patient's heart rate, resulting in the QTc measurement. This is called the corrected QT interval (QTc) and is performed by most 12-lead ECG machines automatically.

2. Count the number of small boxes that make up the QT interval.

3. Multiply this number by 0.04 seconds.

4. Count the number of small boxes that make up the R-R interval (the distance between the R waves).

5. Multiply this number by 0.04 seconds.

6. Calculate the square root of the R-R interval in seconds.

7. Divide the QT interval in seconds by the square root of the R-R interval in seconds.

8. The result is the QTc interval value.

9. The QTc interval value should be one-half of the R-R interval.

- The QT interval should be measured using the same ECG lead.

- An abnormal QT interval:

   ○ A prolonged QT interval indicates a delay in ventricular repolarization. The heart is spending more than normal time depolarized (relative refractory period), making the heart vulnerable to a torsades de pointes (R-On-T phenomenon), resulting in ventricular tachycardia. This can be caused by:

      ▪ Medications such as amiodarone, sotalol, haloperidol, or quinidine

      ▪ Long QT syndrome

      ▪ Hypothyroidism

      ▪ Hypocalcemia

      ▪ Hypomagnesemia

      ▪ Hypothermia

      ▪ Bradyrhythmia

3.9 U Wave

The U wave is a small rounded symmetric wave with an amplitude of <2 mm that is not always present on an ECG graph. The absence of the U wave is not abnormal, nor is the presence of a U wave that is <2 mm. This is commonly seen in patients with slower cardiac rhythms (Figure 3.10).

- Abnormal U wave:

   ○ A U wave ≥2 mm

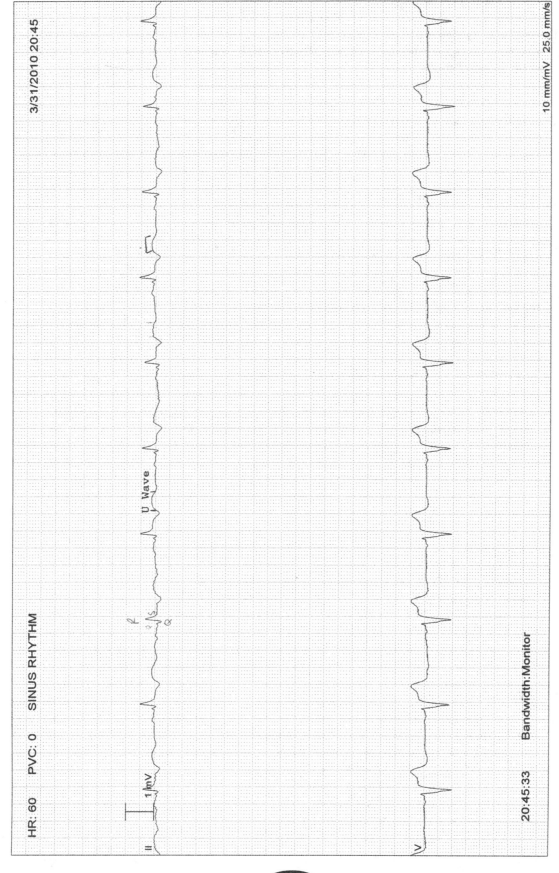

Figure 3.10 The U wave is common in slow cardiac rhythms.

  ○ Caused by:

   ▪ Hypokalemia

   ▪ Hypercalcemia

   ▪ Thyrotoxicosis (a hypermetabolic state or syndrome caused by elevated T3 and T4)

   ▪ Intracranial hemorrhage

Solved Problems

Components of an ECG Tracing

3.1   How many seconds does each large block represent on the ECG graph if the graph paper is moving at a rate of 12 mm/sec?

One large block passes the stylus every 200 ms.

3.2   What is the function of ECG electrodes?

Electrodes placed on the patient's body detect electrical changes in the electrophysiology of cardiac muscle, which is transmitted through wires to the electrocardiograph.

3.3   How are electrophysiologic changes in cardiac muscle represented in an ECG graph?

Electrical changes cause the ECG stylus to move vertically on the graph paper, drawing a line image that reflects the corresponding electrical changes in the electrophysiology of cardiac muscle. This image is recognized as the PQRST sequence that occurs over a measurable time frame.

P Wave

3.4   What does the P wave represent?

The P wave is the first deflection of the isoelectric line and starts when there is electrical activity at the SA node, signifying atrial depolarization.

3.5   What is the normal height of a P wave?

No more than 2.5 mm in height (two and a half small boxes) because the atrium is a smaller muscle mass requiring less voltage to depolarize cells than with the ventricles.

3.6   What is measured by the P wave?

The P wave measures the duration of atrial depolarization.

3.7   What is the normal duration of atrial depolarization?

No more than 0.10 seconds.

3.8   What might be indicated by a tall, peaked P wave?

A tall, peaked P wave indicates right atrial enlargement (RAE) as seen in severe pulmonary diseases such as COPD, asthma, congenital heart disease, and acute pulmonary embolism.

3.9   What might be indicated in an inverted or absent P wave?

An inverted or absent P wave indicates that the initial electrical impulse is originating other than by the SA node (ectopic in nature) and is seen in junctional rhythms.

PR Interval

3.10   What does the PR interval represent?

The PR interval represents the time the electrical impulse takes to travel to the ventricles after atrial repolarization.

3.11   What is the normal duration of the PR interval?

The normal duration of the PR interval is between 0.12 and 0.20 seconds.

3.12   What might be indicated if the duration of the PR interval is <0.12 seconds?

- A shorter path was taken to send the impulse to the ventricles.

- An accessory pathway was used to send the impulse other than through the AV node, such as in Wolff-Parkinson-White disease.

- The impulse begins from a site other than the SA node (ectopic site) that is closer than the SA node is to the AV node.

3.13   What might be indicated if the duration of the PR interval is >0.20 seconds?

- Slower conduction of the impulse through the AV node seen in:

  o Toxicity of medication that slows conduction (i.e., digitalis toxicity)

  o Aging

  o Hypothyroidism

  o First-degree heart block rhythm

3.14   What electrical impulse is being received by the ECG during the PR interval?

None. The PR interval is represented by the isoelectric line.

QRS Complex

3.15   What does the QRS complex represent?

The QRS complex is a three-wave deflection of the isoelectric line that traces the electrical impulse after leaving the AV node and travels through the bundle of His, resulting in ventricular depolarization.

3.16   Why is it sometimes difficult to locate the end of the QRS complex?

It is sometimes difficult to locate the end of the S wave because of variations in the elevation/depression of the ST segment.

3.17   How do you differentiate between the QRS complex and the isoelectric line of the ST segment?

The QRS complex is identified by the width of the QRS line image on the graph. The isoelectric line is thicker (fatter) than the QRS line image on the graph.

3.18   What is R′?

This is called an R prime, indicating that the QRS complex has more than one R wave.

3.19   What is S′?

This is called an S prime, indicating that the QRS complex has more than one S wave.

3.20   What does a notched QRS complex indicate?

A notched QRS complex indicates a bundle branch block where conduction through the bundle branches is blocked.

3.21   What is indicated by a QRS complex >0.12 mm?

Widened QRS (>0.12 mm) indicates early depolarization of the ventricles caused either by the impulse following an accessory pathway other than through the AV node or the initiating impulse is beginning in the ventricles (ectopic beat).

The ST Segment

3.22   What might be indicated by a concave elevation >2 mm?

A nonacute myocardial infarction (AMI) relating to benign early ventricular repolarization or pericarditis might be indicated by a concave elevation >2 mm.

3.23   What is indicated by a horizontal elevation >1 mm?

A myocardial infarction is indicated by a horizontal elevation >1 mm.

3.24   What is indicated by an elevated ST segment in all leads?

A cause other than myocardial infarction, such as pericarditis, is indicated by an elevated ST segment in all leads.

3.25   What is indicated by a generalized tall, peaked T wave?

Hyperkalemia is indicated by a generalized tall, peaked T wave.

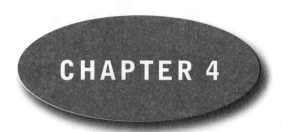

CHAPTER 4

Cardiac Monitoring Equipment and Lead Placement

4.1 Definition

A cardiac monitor is a device that represents the electrophysiology of the heart in a tracing of a line. The tracing forms a straight line called the *isoelectric line* when no electrical activity is detected. Electrical properties of cardiac muscle cause deflection in the isoelectric line.

Wires called *leads* connect the cardiac monitor to transducers called *electrodes* that are strategically placed on the patient's body. A transducer (electrode) is an electrical/mechanical device that detects electrical activity of the heart and translates the activity into electrical waves used by the cardiac monitor to form the tracing.

Three commonly used cardiac monitors are a 12-, 5-, and 3-lead electrocardiograph (ECG) monitor.

1. **A 12-lead electrocardiograph** is a device that produces 12 different tracings on graph paper, enabling the health care provider to record and study the electrophysiology of the heart and offering a 12-view snapshot of the heart. It is ideal for accurate diagnosis of varying degrees and locations of acute coronary syndrome (ACS), such as ischemia vs. infarct. This device should be used during an arrhythmia.

2. **A 3- or 5-lead cardiac monitor** displays the tracing on a screen and is used to study the current electrical activity of the heart over a relatively short time period. These are commonly seen at the bedside, nursing stations, and operating rooms.

3. **Cardiac telemetry** is used in the clinical setting, enabling the patient to ambulate while being monitored. In cardiac telemetry, leads attached to the patient connect to a radio transmitter, which is a small box carried by the patient. The radio transmitter sends electrical waves that represent cardiac activity to a radio transmitter connected to a video cardiac monitor located either at the nurses' station, a central cardiac telemetry unit, or both.

4.2 Waveforms and Current Flow

The lead creates the tracing by measuring the electrical activity of the heart over the lead. Each lead has two electrodes. One electrode is called the positive (+) pole and the other the negative (−) pole. The shape of the waveform depicted in the tracing depends on the placement of the lead related to the path of cardiac electrical activity.

- Electrical activity detected by the positive pole of the lead causes a positive deflection (above the isoelectric line) in the tracing.

- Electrical activity detected by the negative pole results in a negative deflection (below the isoelectric line) in the tracing.

Einthoven's Triangle

Einthoven's triangle (Figure 4.1) is the imagery used to position leads on the patient's body. This is named for Dr. Willem Einthoven, a Dutch physician and physiologist who invented the first practical electrocardiogram in 1903.

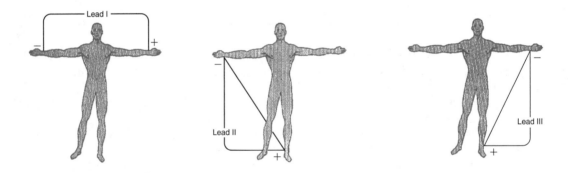

Figure 4.1 Leads are positioned on the body to form Einthoven's triangle.

Einthoven's triangle is an inverted equilateral triangle centered on the patient's chest. Corners of the triangle point to locations where one should place leads on the patient's body. There are three leads, each identified by a number and referred to commonly as the *limb leads*.

1. **Lead I:** This is the top of Einthoven's triangle. The negative pole of the lead is positioned at the patient's right shoulder and the positive pole of the lead is positioned at the patient's left shoulder. This generates a positive deflection in the tracing as current flows right to left (negative to positive) and is helpful in detecting atrial arrhythmias.

2. **Lead II:** This is the right side of Einthoven's triangle. The negative pole of the lead is positioned at the patient's right arm and the positive pole of the lead is positioned at the patient's right leg. This generates a positive deflection in the tracing as current flows from the right arm to the right leg and is helpful in detecting atrial and sinus node arrhythmias.

3. **Lead III:** This is the left side of Einthoven's triangle. The negative pole of the lead is positioned at the patient's left arm and the positive pole of the lead is positioned at the patient's left leg. This generates a positive deflection in the tracing as current flows from the left arm to the left leg and is helpful in detecting inferior wall myocardia infarction.

Augmented Limb Leads

Augmented limb leads are used to enhance tracings of small electrical waveforms of cardiac electrical activity. Augmented limb leads have one electrode, which is a positive electrode called unipolar. The cardiac monitor uses the wave detected by these leads to manipulate information from the poles of the other leads, resulting in a clearer image of small waveforms.

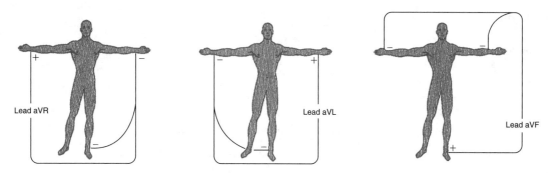

Figure 4.2 Augment limb leads detect small electrical cardiac activity.

Augmented limbs leads are:

- **aVR:** Augmented voltage right arm and positioned on the right arm
- **aVL:** Augmented voltage left arm and positioned on the left arm
- **avF:** Augmented voltage left leg and position on the left leg

Six Precordial Leads

Six precordial leads (Figure 4.3) are placed on the patient's chest. These are single electrode leads, which are positive (unipolar) because of proximity to the heart; these leads do not need augmentation.

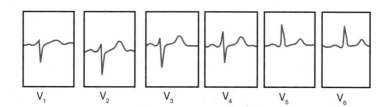

Figure 4.3 Precordial leads are placed on the chest of the patient.

Six precordial leads are identified by their position on the chest:

- **V1 to V2:** Anteroseptal
- **V3 to V4:** Anterior
- **V5 to V6:** Anterolateral

4.3 Electrodes

Electrodes must be placed on the patient properly for them to correctly detect cardiac electrical activity. Improper placement of electrodes can cause artifacts. An artifact is an abnormal variation in the waveform not caused by cardiac electrical activity.

Attaching Electrodes

The initial step in attaching electrodes to the patient is to prepare the skin at the electrode site. This is done by the following method.

- Shave hair from the site.
- Clean the site with alcohol or an acetone pad to remove oil from the skin.
- Abrade (rub) the area with 2 × 2 inch gauze pad to ensure that the skin is clean.
- Clean the site with tincture of benzoin if the patient is sweating, which is common if the patient was administered pain medication.
- Attach the lead to the electrode. It is usually uncomfortable for the patient if the lead is attached to the electrode after the electrode is positioned on the patient's skin.
- Peel back the electrode cover from the gel adhesive pad of the electrode.
- Apply the electrode to the electrode site on the patient's skin. Avoid placing electrodes over bony areas because cardiac electrical activity is better detected through tissue and fluid than bone.
- Select the lead that produces the most defined P wave, usually lead II. But consider the patient's clinical relevance to lead II.

4.4 Bedside Monitors

Bedside monitors are used in critical care units, emergency departments, and surgical suites to monitor the patient's cardiac function. These are commonly referred to as *hardware monitors* because the leads directly connect electrodes to the cardiac monitor.

- *Advantages:* Bedside monitors provide an instant view of the patient's cardiac activity, enabling health care providers to immediately intervene if the patient's cardiac function changes.
- *Disadvantages:* The patient is tethered to the bedside monitor, limiting patient activity and requiring the health care team to work around the leads while caring for the patient. In addition, the patient must be placed on a portable cardiac monitor while being transported to another unit.

Five-Lead Bedside Monitors

A five-lead bedside monitor uses five leads, each with a color-coded electrode (see Figure 4.3). It is designed so that the health care team can continuously monitor any two of the five leads at the same time, which should be V1 for patients with no history of dysrhythmia (rhythms originating outside of the SA node). Lead III and

V3 are best for ST segment monitoring when there is no ischemic fingerprint. The five leads measure voltage between the right limb lead and the feet.

- Left arm positioned at the second intercostals space (between ribs) at the midclavicular
- Right arm positioned at the second intercostals space at the midclavicular
- Left leg positioned at the eighth intercostals space at the midclavicular
- Right leg positioned at the eighth intercostals space at the midclavicular
- Chest lead, which is one of six possible leads:

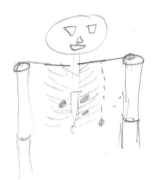

1. V1 positioned at the fourth intercostals space at the right sternal border
2. V2 positioned at the fourth intercostals space at the left sternal border
3. V3 positioned between the fourth and fifth intercostals space
4. V4 positioned at the fifth intercostals space at the left midclavicular line
5. V5 positioned at the fifth intercostals space at the left anterior axillary line
6. V6 positioned at the fifth intercostals space at the midaxillary line

Three-Lead Bedside Monitors

A three-lead bedside monitor uses three leads, each with an electrode. One lead is negative, another is positive, and the third is a ground. The ground lead minimizes interference from artifacts when tracing cardiac activity. The three-lead bedside monitor is typically used with portable bedside monitors to monitor leads I, II, and III.

The three leads are:

1. RA positioned below the clavicle at the second intercostal space at the right midclavicular line
2. LA positioned below the clavicle at the second intercostal space at the left midclavicular line
3. LL positioned on the left lower rib at the eight intercostal space at the left midclavicular line

Leads to Monitor

The lead that should be monitored depends on the patient's clinical picture. Here are commonly used techniques:

- Premature atrial complexes, AV blocks, and sinus abnormalities can be recognized in most leads that display clear P waves. Usually lead I or II is best.
- V1 and V6 are best for differentiating wide QRS rhythms, and monitoring for most arrhythmias. V1 helps distinguish ventricular tachycardia and SVT with aberrancy. SVT with aberrancy is an SVT with an abnormal (aberrant) conduction that takes longer than a normal SVT to travel through the heart, thus causing a wider QRS complex.
- V1 is the best lead to monitor when there is no history of arrhythmia.

- Multiple-lead is better than single-lead monitoring.

- ST-segment monitoring:

  ○ High-risk patients of AMI or ischemia leads III and V3 should be monitored.

  ○ Based on coronary artery involvement, if known, the patient will have ST-segment changes during a cardiac event. These changes are known as an "ischemic fingerprint." If the ischemic finger is known, then use the following leads:

    ▪ I, aVL, V5, and V6 reflect circumflex and the lateral wall

    ▪ II, III, and aVF reflect the right coronary and the inferior wall

    ▪ V1 to V4 reflects the left anterior descending anterior wall

4.5   Telemetry Monitors

Telemetry monitors offer patients and health care providers more freedom than bedside monitors because the leads connect to a wireless transmitter rather than directly to the monitor. The patient is able to move freely and the health care team has little interference from the leads while caring for the patient. However, telemetry monitors are more prone to interference, artifacts, and electrodes inadvertently being removed from position on the patient.

- **Five-Lead Telemetry Monitor:** Uses the same electrode placement as the five-lead bedside monitor. Any of the 12 leads can be monitored, so long as the V1 to V6 leads are properly positioned on the patient's chest.

- **Three-Lead Telemetry Monitor:** Uses the same electrode placement as the five-lead bedside monitor. However, one lead at a time can be monitored.

4.6   Troubleshooting Cardiac Monitors

A common error when interpreting an ECG tracing is that the tracing actually represents electrical activity or movement from external interference and not the patient's heart. It is important to use critical thinking skills when analyzing every tracing because abnormal waveforms on the ECG tracing might be the result of trouble with the cardiac monitor and leads rather than the patient's heart.

Artifacts

An artifact is an abnormal variation in the waveform not caused by cardiac electrical activity that might resemble an abnormal cardiac function. The first reaction to a tracing that indicates an abnormal cardiac function is to verify that the cardiac monitor and leads are properly functioning.

Common causes of artifacts are:

- Patient movement

- Interference from medical equipment connected to the patient

- Poor contact between the electrode and the patient's skin

- A weak signal caused by a poorly functioning electrode, lead, or connector to the cardiac monitor

- Weak battery

False High-Rate Alarms

Cardiac monitors usually have an alarm that sounds when the patient's heart rate increases beyond an acceptable range. This is called a *high-rate alarm*. It is not unusual for an artifact to send a higher than normal electrical signal (high-voltage artifact) to the cardiac monitor that triggers the high-rate alarm. This is called a *false high-rate alarm*.

Some situations that might trigger a false high-rate alarm are:

- Muscle movement

- Head movement

- Tremors in a postoperative patient caused by shivering as a side effect of anesthesia

- Seizure activity

- The use of surgical clippers during an operation

False Low-Rate Alarms

Cardiac monitors usually have an alarm that sounds when the patient's heart rate decreases beyond an acceptable range. This is called a low-rate alarm. It is not unusual for an artifact to send a lower than normal electrical signal (high-voltage artifact) to the cardiac monitor, which triggers the low-rate alarm. This is called a *false low-rate alarm*.

Some situations that might trigger a false low-rate alarm are:

- Weak battery in the cardiac monitor

- Low signal from the electrode or lead or a connector malfunction

- Poor skin contact caused by dried gel on the electrode or sweat at the electrode site

Respiratory Variations

Respiratory variations can affect the cardiac electrical activity that is picked up by electrodes depending on the position of the electrode on the patient's body. This typically results in a wandering isoelectric line (baseline) on the tracing because of exaggerated respiration.

Some patients are abdominal breathers, in which case there is increased movement of the abdomen with each breath. This movement causes electrodes near the abdomen to move, resulting in artifacts.

Patients in respiratory distress also have exaggerated respiration that might affect the electrodes and cause the cardiac monitor to report unusual cardiac activities.

Inspect the Cardiac Monitor

Cardiac monitors and leads can malfunction because of excessive use. It is best to regularly inspect this equipment and repair or replace parts that may become the source of artifacts. By doing so, you address potential problems before they may affect the incorrect interpretation of a tracing.

Areas to inspect are:

- Frayed wires (leads and the power cord)
- Low charge in the cardiac monitor's barriers
- Dried or cracked electrodes

What you can do if you see suspected tracings while monitoring the cardiac function of a patient:

- Reposition electrodes until an acceptable waveform appears in the trace.

- Monitor alternate leads. One lead might be causing the artifact. Other leads will represent actual cardiac activity.

Solved Problems

Cardiac Monitoring

4.1   What is an electrode?

An electrode is an electrical/mechanical device that detects electrical activity of the heart and translates the activity into electrical waves used by a cardiac monitor to form the tracing.

4.2   What is the difference between a lead and an electrode?

A lead connects one or more electrodes to a cardiac monitor.

4.3   What is cardiac telemetry?

Cardiac telemetry is used in the clinical setting, enabling the patient to ambulate while being monitored. In cardiac telemetry, leads attached to the patient connect to a radio transmitter, which is a small box carried by the patient. The radio transmitter sends electrical waves that represent cardiac activity to a radio transmitter connected to a video cardiac monitor located at the nurses' station, a central cardiac telemetry unit, or both.

Waveforms and Current Flow

4.4   What kinds of electrodes are attached to a lead that has two electrodes?

One electrode is called the positive (+) pole and the other the negative (−) pole.

4.5   In which direction does current flow?

The current flows from negative to positive.

4.6   How does the positive pole affect the ECG tracing?

Electrical activity detected by the positive pole of the lead causes a positive deflection (above the isoelectric line) in the tracing.

4.7   How does the negative pole affect the ECG tracing?

Electrical activity detected by the negative pole results in a negative deflection (below the isoelectric line) in the tracing.

4.8   What is Einthoven's triangle?

Einthoven's triangle is the imagery used to position leads on the patient's body. Einthoven's triangle is an inverted equilateral triangle centered on the patient's chest.   .

4.9   Where is lead I positioned?

Lead I is positioned at the top of Einthoven's triangle. The negative pole of the lead is positioned at the patient's right shoulder, and the positive pole of the lead is positioned at the patient's left shoulder.

4.10   Where is lead II positioned?

Lead II is at the right side of Einthoven's triangle. The negative pole of the lead is positioned at the patient's right arm, and the positive pole of the lead is positioned at the patient's right leg.

4.11   Where is lead III positioned?

Lead III is at the left side of Einthoven's triangle. The negative pole of the lead is positioned at the patient's left arm, and the positive pole of the lead is positioned at the patient's left leg.

4.12   What is the current flow of lead II?

The current of lead II flows from the right arm to the right leg.

4.13   What is lead III helpful in detecting?

Lead III is helpful in detecting inferior wall myocardial infarction.

4.14   What is lead I helpful in detecting?

Lead I is helpful in detecting atrial arrhythmias.

4.15   What is the purpose of augmented limb leads?

Augmented limb leads are used to enhance tracings of small electrical waveforms of cardiac electrical activity.

4.16   What makes an augmented limb lead different from lead I?

Augmented limb leads have one electrode.

4.17   What is the electrode called on an augmented limb lead?

The electrode on an augmented limb lead is called unipolar.

4.18   What are precordial leads?

Precordial leads are leads placed on the patient's chest to enhance the tracing.

Electrodes

4.19 How do you attach electrodes to a patient?

- Shave hair from the site.

- Clean the site with alcohol or an acetone pad to remove oil from the skin.

- Abrade (rub) the area with a 2 × 2 inch gauze pad is ensure the skin is clean.

- Clean the site with tincture of benzoin if the patient is sweating, which is common if the patient was administered pain medication.

- Attach the lead to the electrode. It is usually uncomfortable for the patient if the lead is attached to the electrode after the electrode is positioned on the patient's skin.

- Peel back the electrode cover from the gel adhesive pad of the electrode.

- Apply the electrode to the electrode site on the patient's skin. Avoid placing electrodes over bony areas because cardiac electrical activity is better detected through tissue and fluid than bone.

Bedside Monitors

4.20 What are disadvantages of bedside monitors?

The patient is tethered to the bedside monitor, limiting patient activity and requiring the health care team to work around the leads while caring for the patient. In addition, the patient must be placed on a portable cardiac monitor while being transported to another unit.

4.21 What is the purpose of the ground lead in a three-lead bedside monitor?

The ground lead minimizes interference from artifacts when tracing cardiac activity.

Troubleshooting

4.22 What is an artifact?

An artifact is an abnormal variation in the waveform not caused by cardiac electrical activity that might resemble an abnormal cardiac function.

4.23 What are common causes of artifacts?

Common causes of artifacts are patient movement, interference from medical equipment connected to the patient, poor contact between the electrode and the patient's skin, and a weak signal caused by a poorly functioning electrode, lead, or connector to the cardiac monitor.

4.24 What might trigger a false high-rate alarm?

Muscle movement, head movement, tremors in the postoperative patient caused by shivering as a side effect of anesthesia, seizure activity, and the use of surgical clippers during an operation might trigger a false high-rate alarm.

4.25 What should be examined when inspecting a cardiac monitor?

When inspecting a cardiac monitor, look for frayed wires (leads and the power cord), check for low charge in the cardiac monitor's barriers, and examine for dried or cracked electrodes.

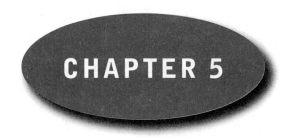

CHAPTER 5

Reading an Electrocardiograph

5.1   Definition

Electrodes that are strategically placed on the patient's body detect electrical impulses from cardiac muscle. Impulses travel through leads into the cardiac monitor where impulses are represented in a tracing that appears on a video screen or drawn by a stylus on ECG (electrocardiograph) graph paper.

In the absence of an electrical impulse, the tracing appears as an isoelectric line (flat line). Cardiac impulses cause an up or down deflection of the isoelectric line. The tracing moves horizontally across the screen (bedside monitor) or ECG graph paper at a rate of 12 mm/sec.

The patient's cardiac function is analyzed by measuring both the height (deflection) from the isoelectric line and the width of the wave (duration of the deflection).

5.2   ECG Graph Paper   *1 small = 0.04 sec   1 lg = 5 small = 0.2 sec*

The ECG graph paper is divided into a grid of small and large boxes, each a specific size, thereby making it relatively simple to measure the tracing (Figure 5.1).

- **Small Box:** The small box is 1 mm square in size and takes 0.04 seconds to pass under the stylus.

- **Large Box:** The large box is comprised of five small boxes. Each large box is 5 mm square and takes 0.20 seconds to pass under the stylus.

5.3   Analyzing Cardiac Rhythm

Electrical activity of the patient's heart is studied by measuring the waveform tracing on the ECG graph. A minimum of 30 large boxes is required to analyze the cardiac rhythm. This is equivalent to six seconds of recording. Three-second marks at the top of the ECG graph paper make it easy to measure recording time.

30 × .2 = 6.0 sec of recorded time

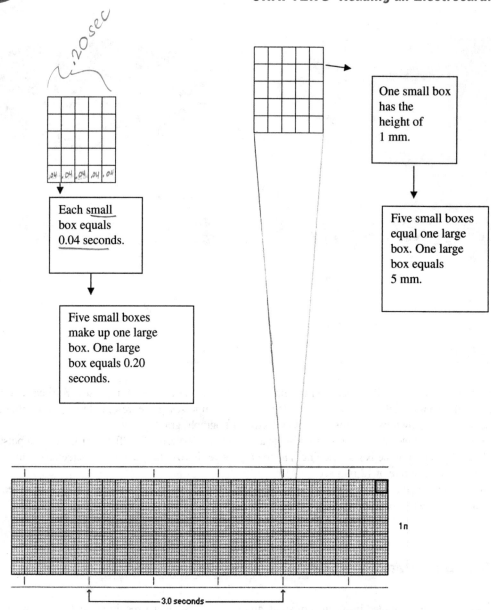

Figure 5.1 Measuring the wave tracing is simple because the ECG graph is divided into a grid.

- Analyze every beat in the six-second strip. Do not take short cuts.
- If the one rhythm converts to another on the same strip, then analyze it as two separate rhythms.

Steps in Analyzing Cardiac Rhythm

There are five characteristics of the tracing used to assess the patient's cardiac rhythm:

1. **Regularity:** Regularity is the recurrence of the same waveform. The waveform should be the same throughout the six-second recording.

2. **Heart Rate:** The heart rate should be between 60 and 100 bpm.

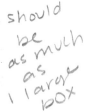

3. **P Wave:** The P wave's height and duration should be within the normal range.

4. **PR Interval:** The PR interval should be within the normal range (0.12 to 0.20 seconds).

5. **QRS Complete:** The QRS complex's height and duration should be within the normal range (0.04 to 0.10 seconds).

PR should be much as as 1 large box

5.4   Regularity

Cardiac electrical activity is regular if the heart is functioning normally. Electrical activity is the same for each heartbeat; therefore, each waveform should be the same on the ECG. This is referred to as *regularity of the tracing*.

Regularity of the rhythm is measured by using either an ECG caliper or an index card. An ECG caliper is a ruler with preset calibrations used to measure waveforms on the ECG graph. An index card can also be used if an ECG caliper is not available by marking the R wave on one complex and the R wave on the next complex, and then using these markings to compare the R to R across the ECG strip.

Measuring Regularity

Here is how to measure regularity (Figure 5.2):

1. Begin on the left side of the ECG graph paper.

2. Place the caliper on the first two R waves. Alternatively, place the index card on the first two R waves then mark both positions on the index card.

3. Move the caliper or index card to the next set of R waves. Each set of R waves should line up with the calibrations on the caliper or the markings on the index card.

4. The rhythm is regular if any irregularity is less than three small boxes.

5. Note any irregularity greater than three small boxes because this might be clinically significant.

5.5   Rate   *can do 300 method b/t R-R OR 6 sec R x 10*

The rate of the rhythm is the patient's heart rate. Before analyzing the rate, determine the regularity of the rhythm. Then decide the appropriate method to assess the rate of the tracing.

Measuring Rate

There are two methods used to measure the rate of the rhythm. The first method is used only if the rhythm is regular. The second method is used to make a quick assessment of the heart rate, regardless of the regularity of the rhythm (Figure 5.3).

- Measuring a regular rhythm rate:
  - Count the small boxes between the R waves.
  - Divide 1500 by the sum of the small boxes between the R waves to determine the rate; 1500 is the number of small boxes that passes the stylus in one minute.

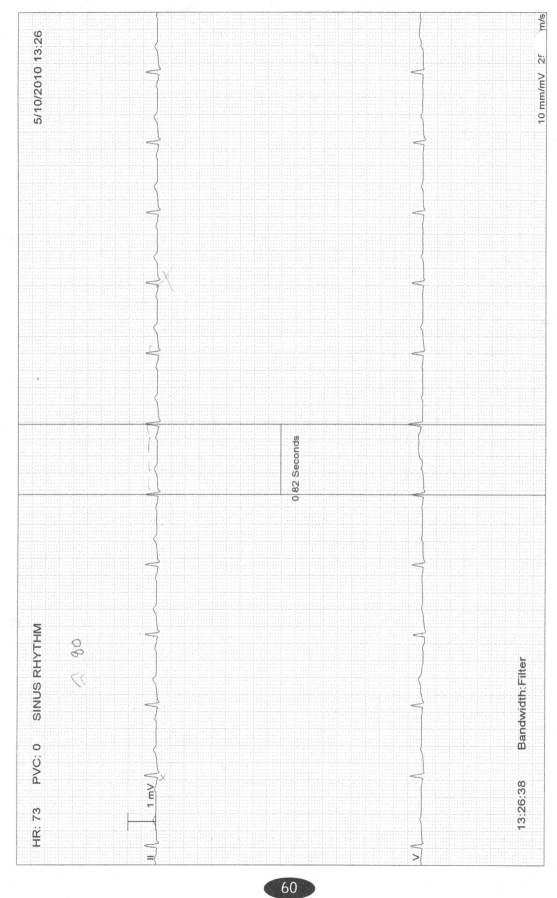

Figure 5.2 Measuring the distance between R waves.

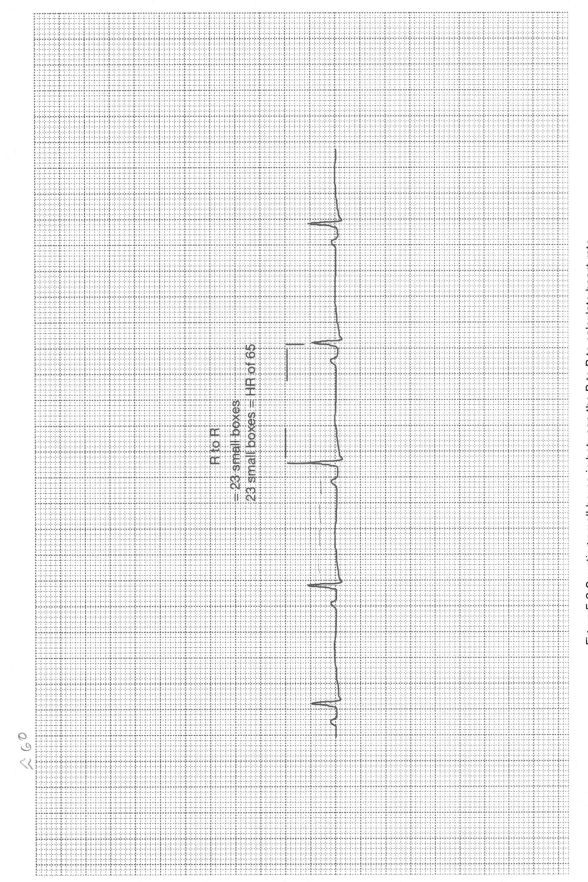

R to R
= 23 small boxes
23 small boxes = HR of 65

Figure 5.3 Counting small boxes in between the R to R to calculate heart rate.

- ○ Alternatively, use the conversion table to find the rate that corresponds to the number of small boxes between the R waves (see Table 5.1).
- Measuring an irregular or regular rhythm rate:
  - ○ Count the number of R waves in the six-second strip.
  - ○ Multiply the number of R waves by 10 to arrive at the rate.
  - ○ If the rhythm is split equally into three-second strips, multiply the rate by 20.

TABLE 5.1 Conversion Table for Heart Rate (HR)

# OF SMALL BOXES	HR/MIN	# OF SMALL BOXES	HR/MIN	# OF SMALL BOXES	HR/MIN
5	300	26	58	50	30
6	250	27	56	60	25
7	214	28	54	70	20
8	188	29	52	80	20
9	167	30	50	90	17
10	150	31	48	100	14
11	136	32	47		
12	125	33	45		
13	115	34	44		
14	107	35	43		
15	100	36	42		
16	94	37	41		
17	88	38	40		
18	84	39	39		
19	79	40	38		
20	75	41	37		
21	72	42	36		
22	68	43	35		
23	65	44	34		
24	63	45	33		
25	60				

5.6   P Wave

The P wave is the first waveform traced and represents the impulse at the SA node, resulting in atrial depolarization (contraction). The initial assessment of the P wave is to determine if the P wave is within normal boundaries. If it is not, then further analysis is performed.

Measuring the P Wave

There are five characteristics that are examined when measuring the P wave in a tracing. Further analysis is required if any of these characteristics do not appear in the tracing.

- Are there P waves in the tracing?
    - ○ The P wave begins when the stylus leaves the isoelectric line and ends when the stylus returns to the isoelectric line.
- Is there one P wave for every QRS complex?
- Is the P wave upright and rounded?
- Is each P wave in the tracing identical?

5.7 PR Interval

The PR interval (PRI) (Figure 5.4) is the period between the end of the P wave and the beginning of the QRS complex, and represents the time the electrical impulse takes to travel to the ventricles after atrial repolarization.

Measuring the PR Interval

Here is how to measure the PR interval:

1. Count the number of small boxes from the beginning of the P wave to the beginning of the QRS complex.

2. Multiply the sum by 0.04 to derive the size of the PR interval.

3. The normal PR interval is between 0.12 to 0.20 seconds.

5.8 QRS Complex

The QRS complex has three waveforms that trace the electrical impulse after leaving the AV node and travel through the bundle of His, resulting in ventricular depolarization.

Measuring the QRS Complex

Here is how to measure the QRS complex (Figure 5.5):

1. Count the number of small boxes between the beginning of the Q wave and the end of the S wave. The QRS line is thinner than the isoelectric line, which makes it easy to distinguish where one begins and the other ends.

2. Multiply the sum by 0.04 seconds to arrive at the measurement of the QRS complex.

3. The normal QRS wave is between 0.04 to 0.10 seconds.

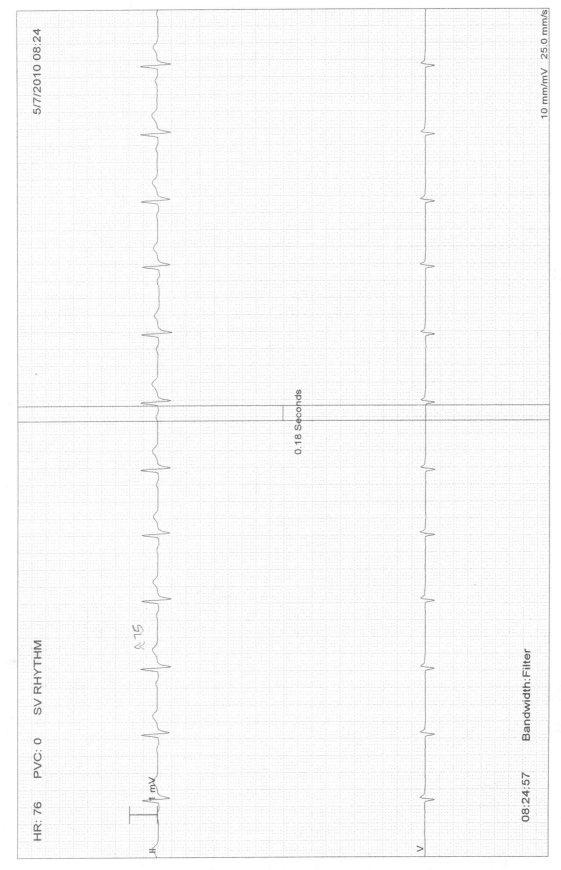

Figure 5.4 The PR interval is measured from the beginning of the P wave to the beginning of the QRS complex.

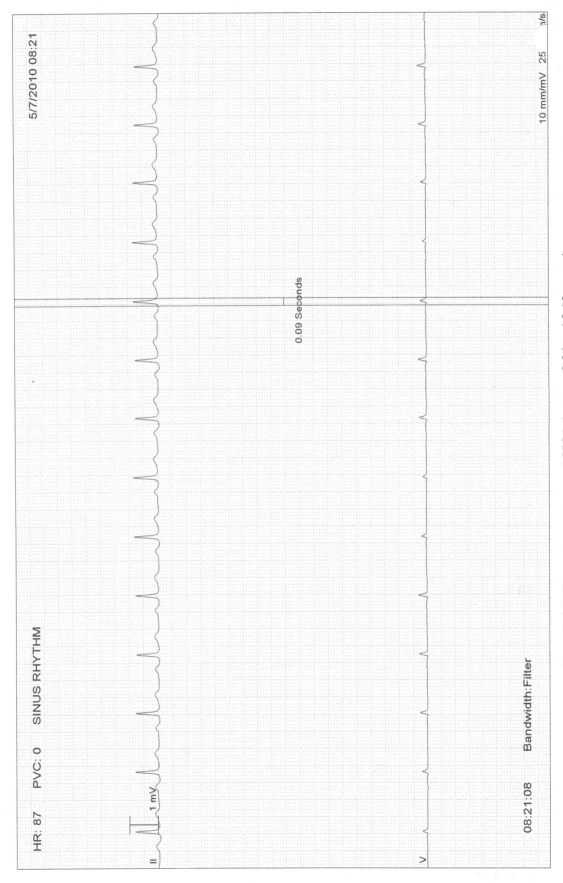

Figure 5.5 QRS measurement—normal QRS is between 0.04 and 0.10 seconds.

Solved Problems

5.1   What is the regularity of Figure 5.6?

Regularity: Irregular

5.2   What is the rate of Figure 5.6?

Rate: 89 bpm

5.3   What is the P wave of Figure 5.6?

P wave: 0

5.4   What is the PR interval of Figure 5.6?

PR interval: 0 seconds

5.5   What is the QRS complex of Figure 5.6?

QRS complex: 0.12 seconds

5.6   What is the regularity of Figure 5.7?

Regularity: Regular

5.7   What is the rate of Figure 5.7?

Rate: 63 bpm

5.8   What is the P wave of Figure 5.7?

P wave: Sinus

5.9   What is the PR interval of Figure 5.7?

PR interval: 0.20 seconds

5.10   What is the QRS complex of Figure 5.7?

QRS complex: 0.08 seconds

5.11   What is the regularity of Figure 5.8?

Regularity: Regular

5.12   What is the rate of Figure 5.8?

Rate: 65 bpm

5.13   What is the P wave of Figure 5.8?

P wave: Sinus

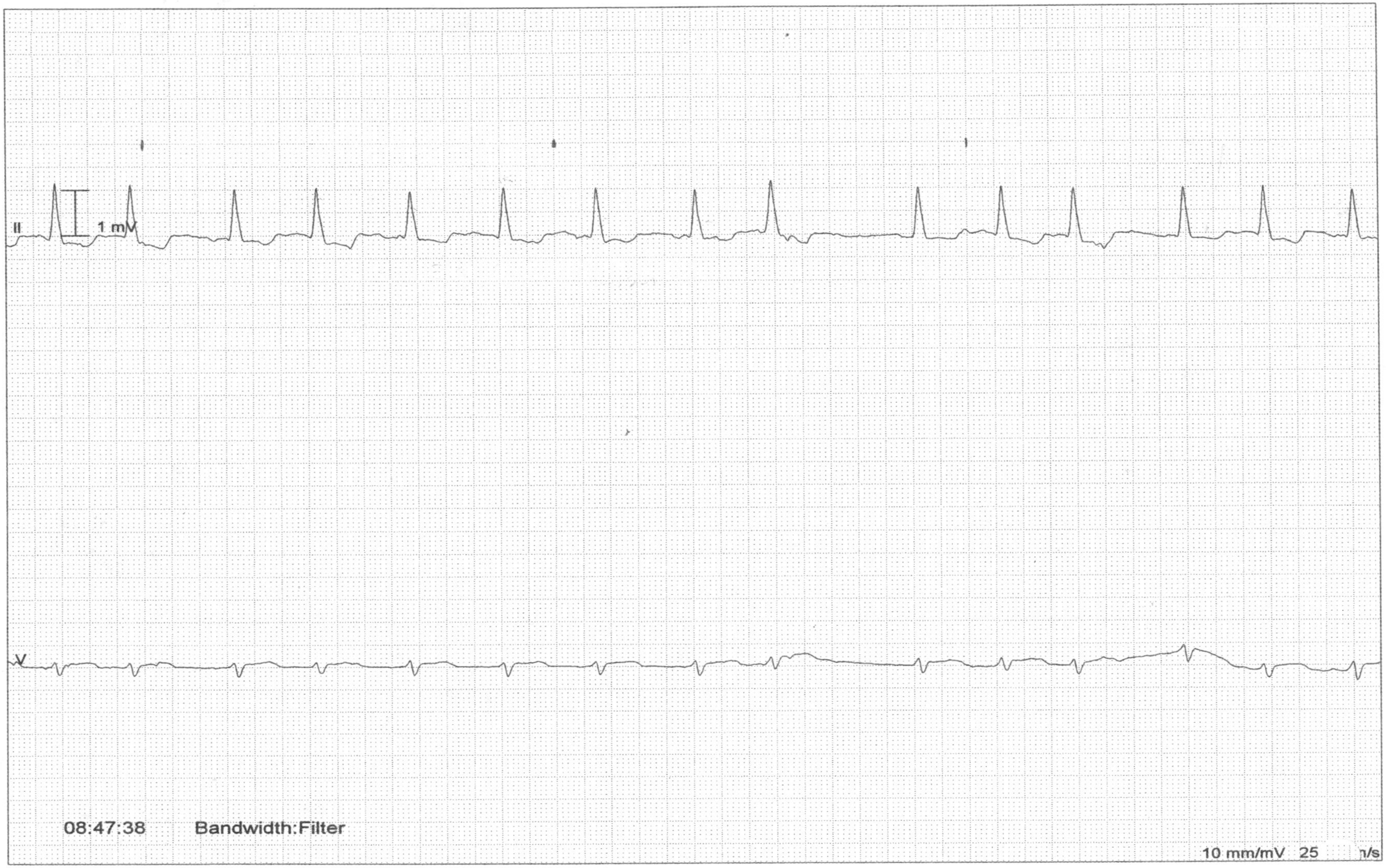

08:47:38   Bandwidth:Filter

10 mm/mV   25   1/s

Figure 5.6

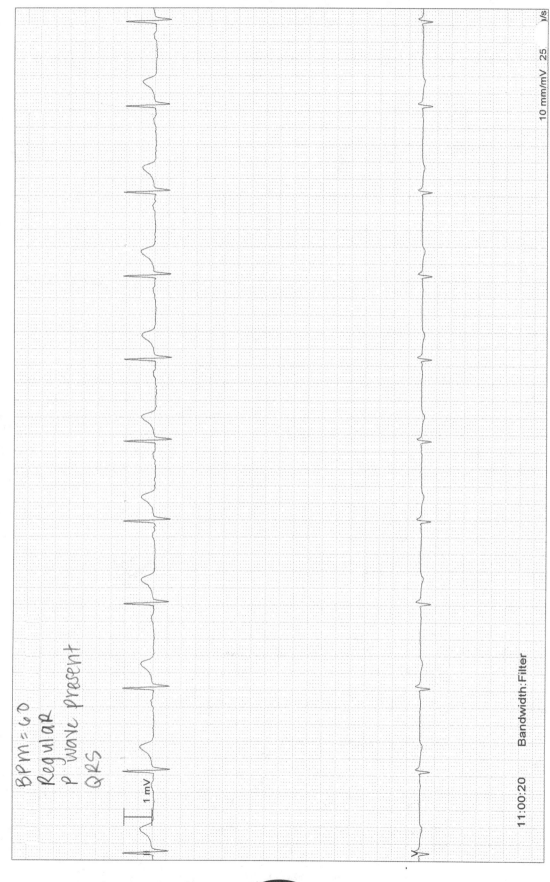

BPM=60
Regular
P wave present
QRS

1 mv

$\frac{60}{ST\ 300}$

11:00:20   Bandwidth:Filter

10 mm/mV   25

Figure 5.7

68

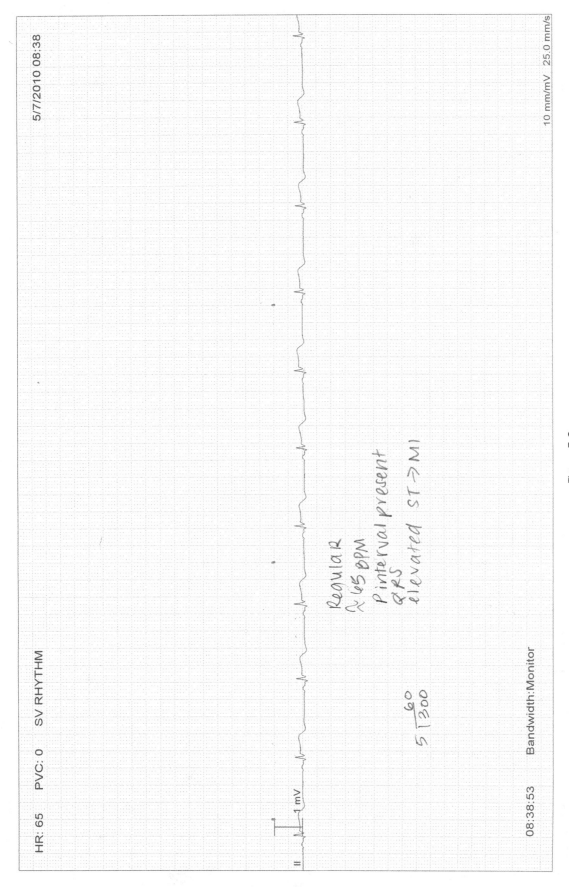

Figure 5.8

5.14   What is the PR interval of Figure 5.8?

PR interval: 0.16 seconds

5.15   What is the QRS complex of Figure 5.8?

QRS complex: 0.08 seconds

5.16   What is the regularity of Figure 5.9?

Regularity: Regular

5.17   What is the rate of Figure 5.9?

Rate: 47 bpm

5.18   What is the P wave of Figure 5.9?

P wave: Sinus

5.19   What is the PR interval of Figure 5.9?

PR interval: 0.20 seconds

5.20   What is the QRS complex of Figure 5.9?

QRS complex: 0.08 seconds

5.21   What is the regularity of Figure 5.10?

Regularity: Irregular

5.22   What is the rate of Figure 5.10?

Rate: 60 bpm

5.23   What is the P wave of Figure 5.10?

P wave: Sinus

5.24   What is the PR interval of Figure 5.10?

PR interval: 0.16 seconds

5.25   What is the QRS complex of Figure 5.10?

QRS complex: 0.06 seconds

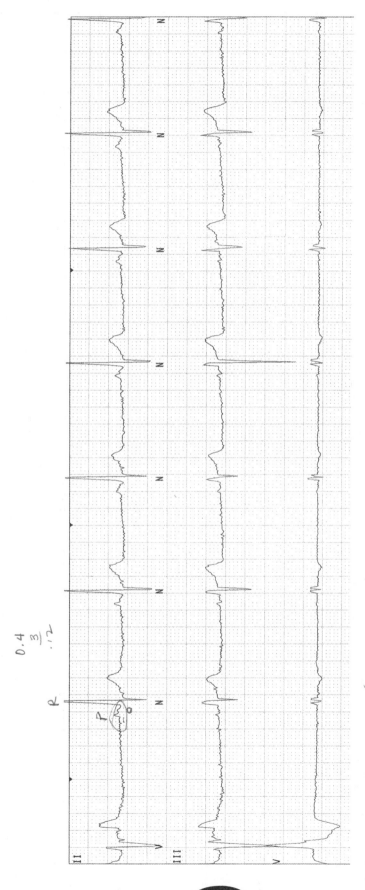

Figure 5.9

Regular ✓
BPM ≈ 50 BPM ✓
P wave Present ✓ sinus
QRS ≈ .12 – .20

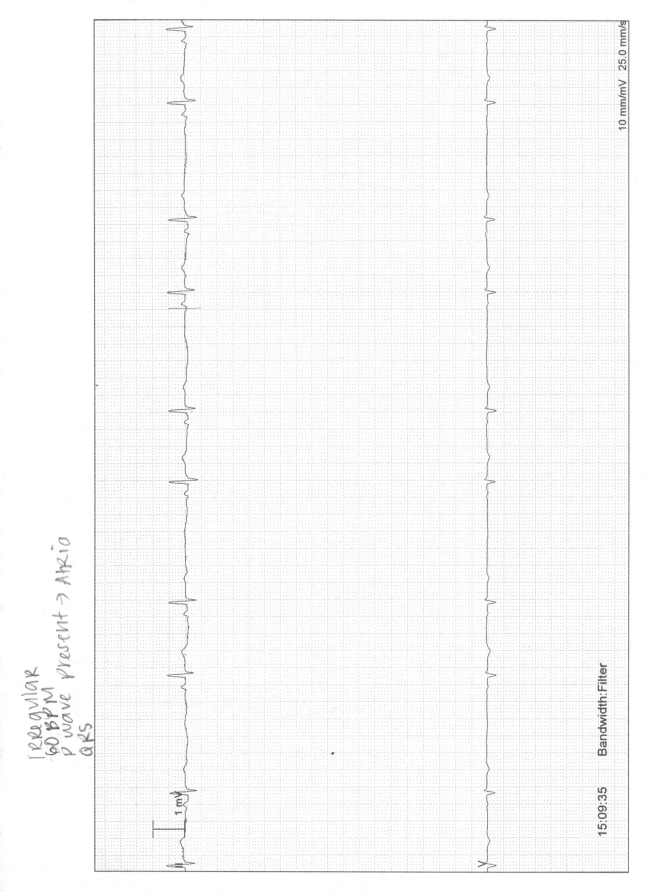

Irregular
60 BPM
P wave present → Atrio
QRS

1 mV

15:09:35   Bandwidth:Filter

10 mm/mV   25.0 mm/s

Figure 5.10

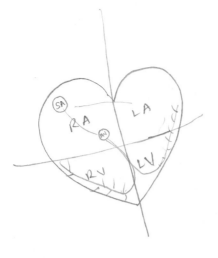

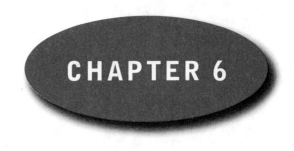

CHAPTER 6

Sinus Rhythms

6.1 Definition

A normally functioning heart generates predictable electrical activity. When measured by an ECG tracing this activity is called a normal sinus rhythm (NSR). Any variation of the normal sinus rhythm is called sinus arrhythmia and might indicate a cardiac malfunction or an artifact that has no relevance to cardiac function.

Normal Sinus Rhythm

Normal sinus rhythm (Figure 6.1) on an ECG means that the cardiac cycle is following the normal intrinsic cycle synchronizing contraction of the atriums with the ventricles, causing pumping action, and forcing blood to circulate throughout the body.

The electrical impulse:

- Initiates at the SA node   60-100
- Travels through the internodal pathway
- Moves into the left atrium via the pathway called Bachmann's bundle resulting in atrial contraction
- Enters the AV node
- Travels into the bundle of His
- Moves through the bundle branches
- Travels into the Purkinje fibers, causing the ventricles to contract

Measuring Normal Sinus Rhythm

Normal sinus rhythm is defined by a range of measurements of the waveforms on the tracing. The tracing displays a normal sinus rhythm if the waveform is within the following ranges:

- **Rate:** 60 to 100 bpm
- **P Wave:** One P wave for every QRS complex. The P wave is upright and rounded in lead II.

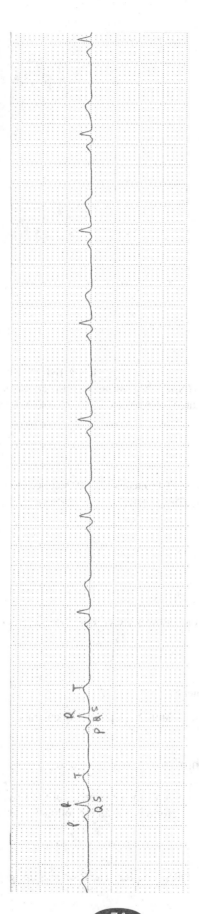

Figure 6.1 A cardiac cycle that follows the normal intrinsic cycle is called a normal sinus rhythm.

[handwritten: 3 small, 5 small - 1 big]

- **PR Interval:** 0.12 to 0.20 seconds
- **QRS Complex:** 0.04 to 0.10 seconds

6.2   Sinus Arrhythmia

In describing the cardiac cycle, the term *sinus* means that the impulse initiates at the SA node. If the impulse follows the normal path to depolarize/repolarize the atria and ventricles, then the cardiac cycle is called a *normal sinus rhythm*. However, the impulse might follow an abnormal path because of cardiac disease, resulting in an irregular sinus rhythm (Figure 6.2). This is referred to as *sinus arrhythmia*. Table 6.1 shows the criteria for normal sinus rhythm and sinus arrhythmia.

6.3   Sinus Bradycardia

Sinus bradycardia (Figure 6.3) is a sinus arrhythmia in which the impulse from the SA node discharges at a slower than normal rate, resulting in a slow heart rate.

Measuring Sinus Bradycardia

[handwritten: Sinus Bradycardia 40-60bpm]

The following are characteristics of sinus bradycardia:

- **Rate:** 40 to 60 bpm
    - **P Wave:** One P wave for every QRS complex. (The P wave is upright and rounded in lead II.)
    - **PR Interval:** 0.12 to 0.20 seconds *[handwritten: 3 little 5 little]*
    - **QRS Complex:** 0.04 to 0.10 seconds

Causes of Sinus Bradycardia

The following are commonly associated with sinus bradycardia:

- **Athletic Training:** Not considered clinically significant.
- **Normal Sleeping:** Not considered clinically significant.
- **Acute Inferior Myocardial Infarction:** Perfusion to the right coronary artery is decreased reducing blood supply to the SA node.
- **Administration of Tissue Plasminogen Activator (tPA) or Streptokinase:** After acute myocardial infarction, the patient may be administered tPA or streptokinase to dissolve the blood clot. Sinus bradycardia can occur either during or after administration of the medication as the blood flow returns. This is referred to as a *reperfusion rhythm*.
- **PNS:** Actions that stimulate the peripheral nervous system (PNS).
- **SNS:** Actions that inhibit the sympathetic nervous system (SNS).

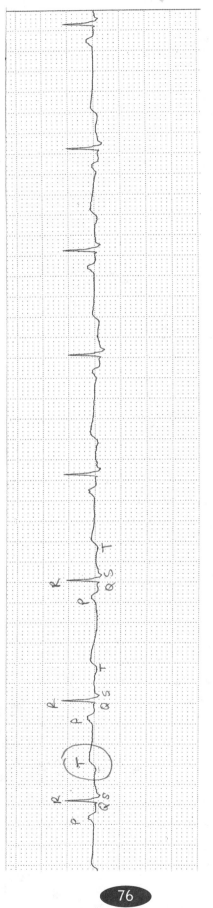

Figure 6.2 An impulse that follows an abnormal path can cause sinus arrhythmia.

Irregular Rhythm
60 BPM
P wave present (sinus)
QRS .12-.20

TABLE 6.1 Criteria for Normal Sinus Rhythm and Sinus Arrhythmia

	RHYTHM	RATE	P WAVES (II)	PR INTERVAL	QRS COMPLEX
Normal sinus rhythm	Regular	60–100	One sinus P wave for each QRS	0.12–0.20	Normal < 0.10 sec
Sinus tachycardia	Regular	100–180	One sinus P wave for each QRS	0.12–0.20	Normal < 0.10 sec
Sinus bradycardia	Regular	40–60	One sinus P wave for each QRS	0.12–0.20	Normal < 0.10 sec
Sinus arrhythmia	Irregular	60–100, but may be <60	One sinus P wave for each QRS	0.12–0.20	Normal < 0.10 sec
Sinus blocks/arrest	Underlying rhythm usually regular, the sudden pause and rate suppression after the event may lend itself to an irregular interpretation. In a block the rhythm will resume on time after the pause. If the rhythm does not resume on time after the pause it is a block.	60–100, but may be <60	One sinus P wave for each QRS, absent during the pause, block and arrest		

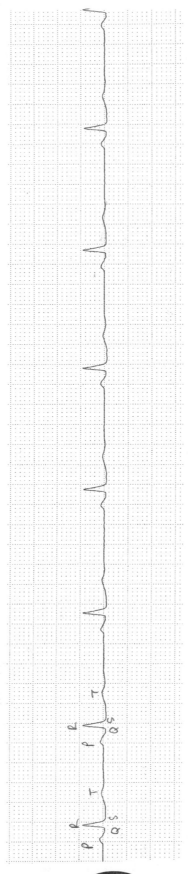

Figure 6.3 A slower impulse causes sinus bradycardia.

Stimulating the PNS and Inhibiting the SNS

The following are common actions that either stimulate the peripheral nervous system or inhibit the sympathetic nervous system, resulting in decreased impulse of the SA node, and causing sinus bradycardia:

- Sleep apnea
- Carotid sinus massage
- Increased intracranial pressure
- Hypothyroidism
- Vomiting
- Ocular pressure
- Sick sinus syndrome (see Sick Sinus Syndrome)
- Valsalva's maneuver (straining)
- Sudden movement to an upright position
- Hypothermia
- Fright
- Medication: Beta blockers, calcium channel blockers, digoxin, and morphine

Treatment for Sinus Bradycardia

Treatment for sinus bradycardia is unnecessary unless the patient exhibits signs or symptoms other than a slow heartbeat such as persistent dizziness, fainting, or fatigue. When the patient becomes symptomatic, the health care provider may treat sinus bradycardia by:

- Asking the patient to cough to decrease the vagal tone
- Administering atropine to inhibit parasympathetic tone and increase SA impulses (see Chapter 12)
- Administering an external electrical stimulus from either a transcutaneous or transvenous pacemaker

6.4   Sinus Tachycardia

Sinus tachycardia (Figure 6.4) is a sinus arrhythmia where the impulse from the SA node discharges at a faster than normal rate resulting in a fast heart rate.

Measuring Sinus Tachycardia

The following are characteristics of sinus tachycardia:

- Sinus tachycardia begins and ends gradually.
- **Rate:** 100 to 180 beats per minute
- **P Wave:** One P wave for every QRS complex. (The P wave is upright and rounded in lead II.)

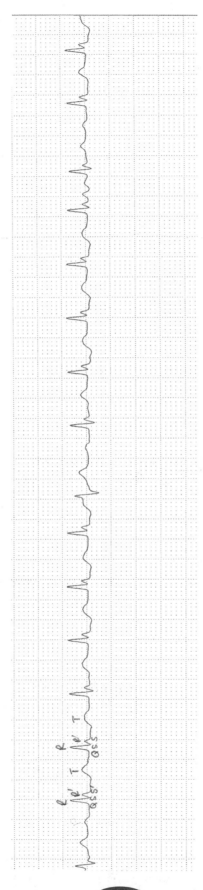

Figure 6.4 A faster impulse causes sinus tachycardia.

- **PR Interval:** This is difficult to measure because of the increased heart rate.
- **QRS Complex:** 0.04 to 0.10 seconds.

Causes of Sinus Tachycardia

The following are commonly associated with sinus tachycardia:

- **Exercise:** Not considered clinically significant.
- **Normal Increased Demand for Blood Flow:** This is not considered clinically significant if the heart rate returns to normal sinus rhythm when demand for blood flow decreases.
- **Acute Myocardial Ischemia:** Decreased perfusion of blood to cardiac muscles increases the demand for oxygen to the heart, resulting in sinus tachycardia.
- **Cardiac Muscle Damage from an Acute Myocardial Infarction:** Damaged cardiac muscle results in decreased perfusion of blood to the heart, signaling a need to increase oxygen to the heart, and resulting in persistent sinus tachycardia.
- **Persistent Sinus Tachycardia:** There is decreased diastole. Diastole occurs when the heart fills with blood. This results in decreased stroke volume and decreased cardiac output, aggravating the myocardial infarction and increasing cardiac muscle damage.
- Actions that inhibit the peripheral nervous system (PNS).
- Actions that stimulate the sympathetic nervous system (SNS).

Inhibiting the PNS and Stimulating the SNS

The following are common actions that either inhibit the parasympathetic nervous system or stimulate the sympathetic nervous system, resulting in increased impulse of the SA node and causing sinus tachycardia:

- Exercise
- Anxiety
- Fever
- Pain
- Anemia
- Hypoxia
- Hypovolemia
- Hypotension
- Myocardial ischemia
- Heart failure
- Alcohol intoxication
- Alcohol withdrawal
- Caffeine
- Smoking

- Pulmonary embolism
- Shock
- Medication:
  - Atropine decreases the vagal tone, thus inhibiting the peripheral nervous system.
  - Epinephrine, dopamine, tricyclic antidepressants, and cocaine stimulate the sympathetic nervous system.

Treatment for Sinus Tachycardia

The treatment for sinus tachycardia is to deal with the underlying cause rather than the fast heart rate. Once the underlying cause is addressed, the need for increased oxygen is no longer required, and therefore the patient's body adjusts to adequate oxygenation by returning to normal sinus rhythm.

6.5   Sinus Arrest and Exit Block

Sinus arrest (Figure 6.5) and exit block (Figure 6.6) is a sinus arrhythmia in which there is one or more missed impulses from the SA node resulting in a skipped heartbeat. The missed heartbeat may have a short duration causing no symptoms. Long duration might result in hypotension, dizziness, or syncope. After an episode, the heart rate might slow (sinus bradycardia) before returning to a normal sinus rhythm.

There are three types of sinus arrest and exit block:

1. **Sinus Pause:** This lasts less than two cardiac cycles or two R to R intervals.
2. **Sinus Block:** This is equal to two cardiac cycles or two R to R intervals.
3. **Sinus Arrest:** This lasts longer than two cardiac cycles or two R to R cycles.

Measuring Sinus Arrest and Exit Block

How to measure the sinus arrest and exit block:

- Determine the type of sinus arrest and exit block.
  - Measure the number of small blocks between the R waves of two cardiac cycles in the normal sinus rhythm portion of the tracing.
  - Count the number of small blocks between R waves in the break in the rhythm (the missing waveform).
  - If the break is less than the number of small blocks in the two cardiac cycles, then it is a sinus pause.
  - If the break is equal to the number of small blocks in the two cardiac cycles, then it is a sinus block.
  - If the break has more small blocks than the two cardiac cycles, then it is a sinus arrest.
- Determine if the breaks are progressively longer.
  - Count the small boxes between succeeding breaks.
  - Multiply the sum by 0.04 seconds to determine if the duration of the breaks is increasing.

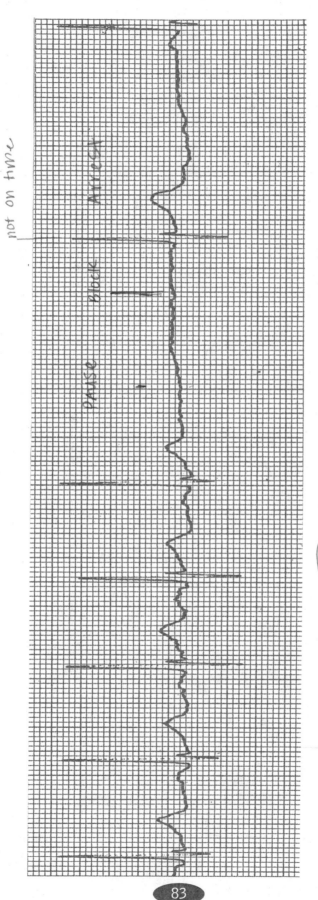

Figure 6.5 A sinus arrest results in a skipped heartbeat. Sixth beat is an escape beat.

Pause
not on time

Block

Arrest

Pause   Arrest

Block

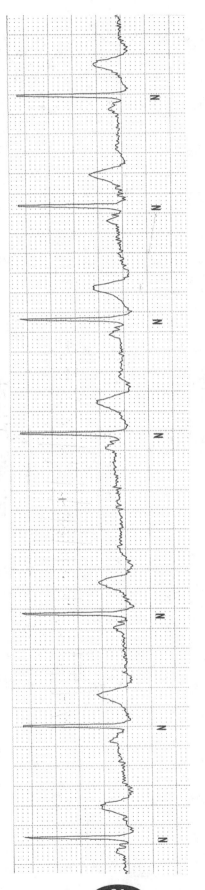

Figure 6.6 A sinus exit block might have no symptoms or the patient might be symptomatic.

Causes of Sinus Arrest and Exit Block

The following are commonly associated with sinus arrest and exit block:

- Increased vagal tone stimulating the peripheral nervous system
- Damage to the SA node
- Hypoxia
- Hyperkalemia
- Medication: Digoxin, beta blockers, or calcium channel blockers

Treatment for Sinus Arrest and Exit Block

Treatment for sinus arrest and exit block is unnecessary unless the patient exhibits signs or symptoms such as persistent hypotension, dizziness, or syncope. When the patient becomes symptomatic, the health care provider may treat sinus arrest and exit block by:

- Asking the patient to cough to decrease the vagal tone
- Administering atropine to inhibit parasympathetic tone and increase SA impulses (see Chapter 12)
- Administering an external electrical stimulus from either a transcutaneous or transvenous pacemaker

6.6   Sick Sinus Syndrome

Sick sinus syndrome, also known as sinus node dysfunction and tachy-brady syndrome, is the failure of the SA node to function properly. Sick sinus syndrome can be the underlying cause of:

- **Sinus Bradycardia:** Slow heart rate
- **Sinus Tachycardia:** Fast heart rate
- **Sinus Arrest and Exit Block:** Missed heartbeats
- **Chronotropic Incompetence:** Inability of the sinus node to react adequately to exercise and metabolic stress

Chronotropic incompetence heart does not speed up or slow down

- **Sinoatrial Exit Block:** A second-degree heart block in which the impulse is unable to leave the SA, not the atrium

Causes of Sick Sinus Syndrome

The following are commonly associated with sick sinus syndrome:

- Age-related changes to the SA node and conduction system that is seen in adults >50 years of age
- Medication: Beta blockers, calcium channel blockers
- Hypothyroidism

- Hyperkalemia

- Medication: Digoxin, beta blockers, or calcium channel blockers

- Malfunction of the autonomic nervous system

Treatment of Sick Sinus Syndrome

Treatment of sick sinus syndrome is unnecessary unless the patient exhibits signs or symptoms of sinus bradycardia, sinus tachycardia, or sinus arrest and exit block. When the patient becomes symptomatic, the health care provider may treat sick sinus syndrome by implanting a permanent pacemaker.

Solved Problems

Normal Sinus Rhythm

6.1 What is normal sinus rhythm?

Normal sinus rhythm on an ECG means that the cardiac cycle is following the normal intrinsic cycle synchronizing contraction of the atriums with the ventricles, causing pumping action that forces blood to circulate throughout the body. The electrical impulse initiates at the SA node, travels through the intermodal pathway, moves into Bachmann's bundle, which causes the atriums to contract, enters the AV node, travels into the bundle of His, and moves through the bundle branches into the Purkinje fibers, which causes the ventricles to contract.

6.2 How is normal sinus rhythm measured?

Normal sinus rhythm is defined by a range of measurements of the waveforms on the tracing. The tracing indicates a normal sinus rhythm if the waveform is within the following ranges:

- **Rate:** 60 to 100 bpm

- **P Wave:** One P wave for every QRS complex. (The P wave is upright and rounded in lead II.)

- **PR Interval:** 0.12 to 0.20 seconds

- **QRS Complex:** 0.04 to 0.10 seconds

Sinus Arrhythmia

6.3 What is sinus arrhythmia?

Any variation of the normal sinus rhythm is called sinus arrhythmia and might indicate a cardiac malfunction or an artifact that has no relevance to cardiac function.

6.4 What do the terms *sinus* in *normal sinus rhythm* and *sinus arrhythmia* mean?

The term *sinus* in describing the cardiac cycle means that the impulse initiates at the SA node. If the impulse follows the normal path to depolarize/repolarize the atria and ventricles, then the cardiac cycle is called *normal sinus rhythm*. However, the impulse might follow an abnormal path because of cardiac disease resulting in an abnormal rhythm. This is referred to as *sinus arrhythmia*.

6.5   What is sinus bradycardia?

Sinus bradycardia is a sinus arrhythmia in which the impulse from the SA node discharges at a slower than normal rate, resulting in a slow heart rate.

6.6   What is the heart rate in sinus bradycardia?

The heart rate in sinus bradycardia is 40 to 60 bpm.

6.7   What is unusual about the P wave and QRS complex in sinus bradycardia?

The P wave and QRS complex are normal.

6.8   What might be the cause of non–clinically significant sinus bradycardia?

The cause of non–clinically significant sinus bradycardia might be athletic training or normal sleeping. Both of these are not considered to be clinically significant.

6.9   What medication might cause sinus bradycardia?

Administration of tissue plasminogen activator (tPA) or streptokinase might cause sinus bradycardia. After a myocardial infarction, the patient may be administered tPA or streptokinase to dissolve the blood clot. Sinus bradycardia can occur either during or after administration of the medication as the blood flow returns. This is referred to as *reperfusion rhythm*.

6.10   How might an acute inferior myocardial infarction cause sinus bradycardia?

Perfusion to the right coronary artery is decreased, reducing blood supply to the SA node.

6.11   How can the peripheral nervous system and sympathetic nervous system cause sinus bradycardia?

Actions that stimulate the peripheral nervous system (PNS) or inhibit the sympathetic nervous system (SNS) can cause sinus bradycardia.

6.12   What actions can stimulate the peripheral nervous system (PNS) or inhibit the sympathetic nervous system (SNS)?

Actions that can stimulate the peripheral nervous system (PNS) or inhibit the sympathetic nervous system (SNS) are sleep apnea, carotid sinus massage, increased intracranial pressure, hypothyroidism, vomiting, ocular pressure, sick sinus syndrome, Valsalva's maneuver (straining), sudden movement to an upright position, hypothermia, and fright.

6.13   What medications can cause sinus bradycardia?

Medications that can cause sinus bradycardia are beta blockers, calcium channel blockers, digoxin, and morphine.

6.14   How would you treat a patient who displays sinus bradycardia on an ECG during a routine physical?

Treatment for sinus bradycardia is unnecessary unless the patient exhibits signs or symptoms other than a slow heartbeat such as persistent dizziness, fainting, or fatigue.

Sinus Tachycardia

6.15   What is sinus tachycardia?

Sinus tachycardia is a sinus arrhythmia in which the impulse from the SA node discharges at a faster than normal rate, resulting in a fast heart rate.

6.16   What are the characteristics of sinus tachycardia on an ECG tracing?

- It begins and ends gradually.
- **Rate:** 100 to 180 bpm.
- **P Wave:** One P wave for every QRS complex. (The P wave is upright and rounded in lead II.)
- **PR Interval:** This is difficult to measure because of the increased heart rate.
- **ST Interval:** Normal, not with elevations or depression from baseline.
- **QRS Complex:** 0.04 to 0.10 seconds.

6.17   What are non–clinically significant causes of sinus tachycardia?

Non–clinically significant causes of sinus tachycardia are exercise, which is not considered clinically significant, and normal increased demand for blood flow, which is not considered clinically significant if the heart rate returns to normal sinus rhythm when demand for blood flow decreases.

6.18   What is the ill effect of persistent sinus tachycardia?

The ill effect of persistent sinus tachycardia is decreased diastole. Diastole occurs when the heart fills with blood. This results in decreased stroke volume and decreased cardiac output, aggravating the myocardial infarction and increasing cardiac muscle damage.

6.19   How does acute myocardial infarction cause sinus tachycardia?

Acute myocardial infarction causes sinus tachycardia by decreasing perfusion of blood to cardiac muscles, which increases the demand for oxygen to the heart and results in sinus tachycardia.

6.20   How can the peripheral nervous system and sympathetic nervous system cause sinus tachycardia?

Actions that inhibit the peripheral nervous system (PNS) or stimulate the sympathetic nervous system (SNS) can cause sinus tachycardia.

6.21   What medications can cause sinus tachycardia?

Atropine can cause sinus tachycardia because it decreases the vagal tone, which inhibits the peripheral nervous system. Epinephrine, dopamine, tricyclic antidepressants, and cocaine can cause sinus tachycardia because they stimulate the sympathetic nervous system.

6.22   What is the treatment for sinus tachycardia?

The treatment for sinus tachycardia is to deal with the underlying cause of sinus tachycardia rather than treating the fast heart rate. Once the underlying cause is addressed, the need for increased oxygen is no longer required; therefore, the patient's body adjusts to adequate oxygenation by returning to normal sinus rhythm.

Sinus Arrest and Exit Block

6.23   What is sinus arrest and exit block?

Sinus arrest and exit block is a sinus arrhythmia in which there is one or more missed impulses from the SA node, resulting in a skipped heartbeat.

6.24   What are the three types of sinus arrest and exit blocks?

- **Sinus Pause:** One cardiac cycle is missing (one beat)

- **Sinus Block:** Two cardiac cycles are missing (two beats)

- **Sinus Arrest:** More than two cardiac cycles are missing (more than two beats)

6.25   How do you measure sinus arrest and exit block?

Measure the number of small blocks between the R waves of two cardiac cycles in the normal sinus rhythm portion of the tracing. Count the number of small blocks between R waves in the break in the rhythm (the missing waveform). If the break is less than the number of small blocks in the two cardiac cycles, it is a sinus pause. If the break is equal to the number of small blocks in the two cardiac cycles, it is a sinus block. If the break has more small blocks than the two cardiac cycles, it is a sinus arrest. Determine the type of sinus arrest and exit block. Determine if the breaks are progressively longer. Count the small boxes between succeeding breaks. Multiply the sum by 0.04 seconds to determine if duration of the breaks is increasing.

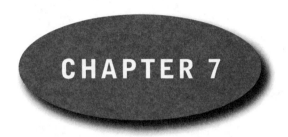

CHAPTER 7

Atrial Arrhythmia

7.1 Definition *ectopic pacemakers*

An arrhythmia is an irregular heartbeat or heart rhythm that is caused when a cardiac cell other than the SA node takes over the role of cardiac pacemaker. This is referred to as an *ectopic pacemaker*. There are three locations on the heart where an ectopic pacemaker is located. The sites of ectopic pacemakers for arrhythmias are:

- **Atrial:** The ectopic pacemaker is located in the atria.
- **Junctional:** The ectopic pacemaker is located at the atrioventricular (AV) junction.
- **Ventricular:** The ectopic pacemaker is located in the ventricles.

Mechanism for an Ectopic Pacemaker

There are three mechanisms responsible for an ectopic pacemaker:

1. **Enhanced/Suppressed Automaticity:** The cardiac cells in the ectopic pacemaker fire at a faster rate than the SA node. As a result, the SA node's automaticity (ability to automatically generate an impulse) is suppressed at the SA node, relinquishing control of the ectopic pacemaker.

2. **Triggered Activity (After Depolarization):** The ectopic pacemaker is triggered to fire an impulse after depolarization and before repolarization, resulting in couplets (two beats) or triplets (three beats) per cardiac cycle. These conditions can occur as a result of:
   - Prolonged QT intervals
   - Bradycardias
   - Hypomagnesemia
   - Hypoxia
   - Digoxin toxicity

3. **Re-entry:** In a normal cardiac cycle, the impulse travels from the SA node in the atria and ends in the ventricles. In re-entry, the impulse travels in a circular path, returning to the SA node. The impulse

continues as long as there is a refractory period within the circle of conduction. The absolute refractory period is the period of time during which cardiac cells are incapable of generating a new impulse. Re-entry is responsible for most atrial flutters (abnormal heart rhythm in the atrium), paroxysmal atrial tachycardia (a regular, fast heartbeat starting in the atria that begins and ends suddenly), and some ventricular tachycardia (a regular, fast heartbeat starting in the ventricles).

7.2　Atrial Arrhythmias

Atrial arrhythmias are arrhythmias that are caused by an ectopic pacemaker located in the atria. Central to atrial arrhythmias is the role of the AV node. The AV node acts as the gatekeeper for the ventricles by protecting the ventricles from responding to every impulse that is generated during atrial fibrillation (afib) and atrial flutter (aflutter).

- **Atrial Fibrillation:** This is the most common arrhythmia involving the atria. Normal impulses generated by the SA node become suppressed by impulses generated by an ectopic pacemaker located in the atria, resulting in the quivering (fibrillating) of the atrial cardiac muscle rather than coordinated contraction (Figure 7.1).
- **Atrial Flutter:** This arrhythmia is caused by a re-entry rhythm of either the right or left atrium caused by an ectopic pacemaker, generating a premature impulse that results in a self-perpetuating loop as the premature impulse moves through atrial cardiac muscle. As a result, the patient feels regular heart palpitations (Figure 7.2).

Atrial Arrhythmias and the ECG

The ECG wave in atrial arrhythmias will show an abnormal P wave because the impulse is conducted through an abnormal pathway from the SA node or an accessory pathway to the AV node. This results in the ventricular rate being slower than the atrial rate as indicated by fewer QRS complexes than P waves. In addition, here are other changes found on the ECG:

- **P Pulmonale:** The point of the P wave is >2.5 mm, indicating an enlarged right atrium.
- **P Mitrale:** The P wave is notched, indicating an enlarged left atrium.
- **Wavy Baseline:** The rhythm is irregular, indicating atrial fibrillation. *SA firing is masked by ectopic impulses*
- **Saw Tooth:** The saw tooth wave indicates atrial flutter. *obtaining impulse from atria other than SA*
- **Inverted P Wave:** The inverted P wave indicates that the ectopic pacemaker is located at the atrioventricular (AV) junction near the AV node.
- **P Wave Superimposed on T Wave:** The P wave superimposed on the preceding T wave indicates paroxysmal atrial tachycardia, which is a regular, fast heartbeat starting in the atria that begins and ends suddenly.

Atrial Arrhythmias Impact

Atrial arrhythmias result in a fast heart rate, which may be tolerated by patients who have no underlying cardiac disease. However, patients who have existing cardiac disease may become symptomatic from the rapid heart rate and decompensate.

　　An increased heart rate decreases diastolic time of the ventricles, resulting in decreased filling and causing the stroke volume to reduce, which decreases the amount of blood that is ejected with each heartbeat. This results

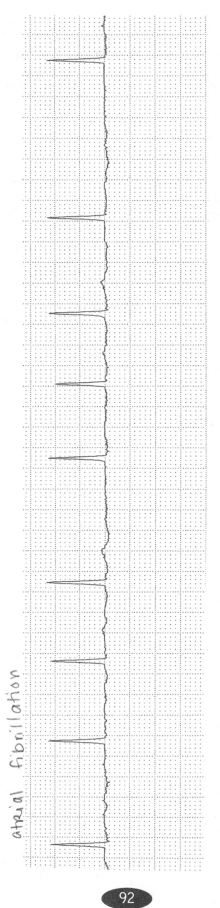

atrial fibrillation

Figure 7.1 Atrial fibrillation with controlled ventricular response.

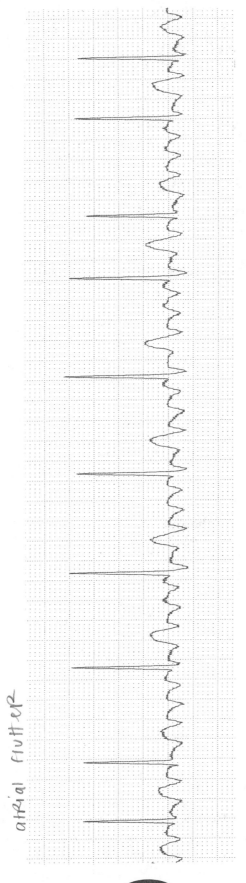

atrial flutter

Figure 7.2 Atrial flutter.

in lower cardiac output and less coronary perfusion because the heart receives its blood supply during the diastole phase. The decrease in coronary perfusion causes an increased heart rate to supply coronary muscles with oxygen. Eventually the myocardium outstrips the supply of oxygenated blood, resulting in the patient becoming symptomatic.

7.3   Premature Atrial Contraction (PAC)

Premature atrial contraction (Figure 7.3) is an impulse before the SA node impulse that originates from one or more atrial ectopic pacemakers that disrupt the normal sinus rhythm. Once the premature impulse reaches the AV node, the conduction path of the impulse follows the same path as the SA node impulse. Frequent premature atrial contractions indicate that the atria are being irritated, which could lead to atrial fibrillation or atrial flutter. Premature atrial contractions may develop the following patterns:

- **Bigeminal:** Every other beat there is a premature atrial contraction.

- **Trigeminal:** Every third beat there is a premature atrial contraction.

- **Quadrigeminal:** Every fourth beat there is a premature atrial contraction.

- **Couplet:** There is a pair of premature atrial contractions.

- **Premature Atrial Tachycardia (PAT):** There are more than three series of premature atrial contractions, which implies that sudden starts and breaks occur by the atrial ectopic pacemaker.

The premature atrial contraction may reach the bundle branches too early—before the bundle branches are fully repolarized. In addition, the impulse from the atrial ectopic pacemaker may travel to the left bundle branch, first causing the left ventricle to depolarize and then travel to the right ventricle, causing the right ventricle to depolarize, resulting in disruption in the coordinated depolarizing of ventricles.

Premature Atrial Contraction and the ECG

The premature atrial contraction is depicted on an ECG as an abnormal P wave that may be hidden in the preceding T wave, in which case the T wave is distorted. The ECG shows an aberrantly conducted PCA, which is a wide or notched QRS complex.

A premature atrial contraction might be difficult to detect on an ECG because the impulse from the ectopic pacemaker follows the same conduction path as the SA node impulse. That is, the QRS complex is the same as that of the SA node impulse.

Adding a further complication, it is confusing to differentiate between premature atrial contractions and premature ventricular contractions. The best way to make the distinction on the ECG is to identify an abnormal P wave and a distorted T wave.

Noncompensatory vs. Compensatory Pauses

Any pause between SA node impulses during PAC is measured from the R wave that occurs immediately before the PAC to the R wave immediately after the PAC.

A noncompensatory pause (Figure 7.4) occurs when early depolarization of the atria resets of the timing of the SA node. The measurement of the pause is less than two R-R intervals in the underlying regular rhythm.

A compensatory pause occurs when the SA node timing is not reset by the PAC. The measurement of the pause is equal to two R-R intervals in the underlying regular rhythm (Figure 7.5). This enables the heart to reset itself or compensate for the extrasystole.

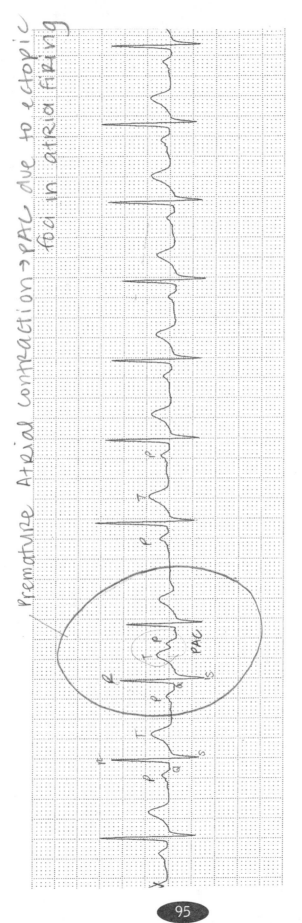

Figure 7.3 Premature atrial contraction at the fourth beat.

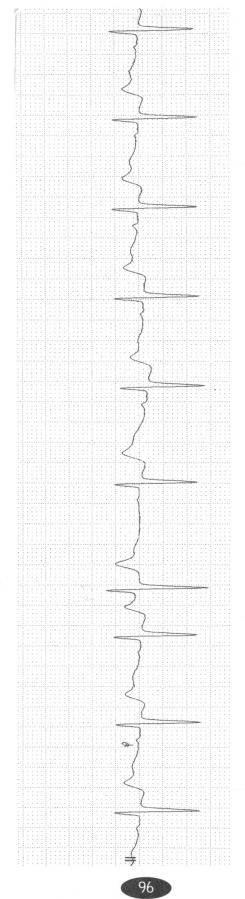

Figure 7.4 PAC with noncompensatory pause. Pause is <2 R-R intervals.

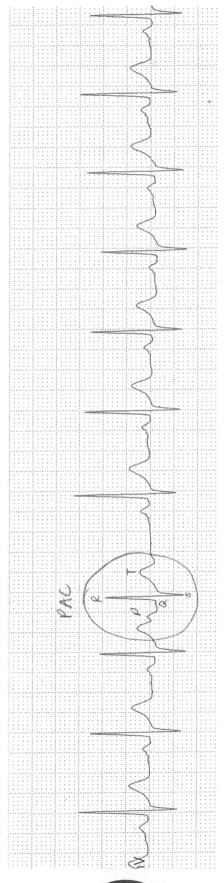

Figure 7.5 PAC with compensatory pause. Pause is equal to two R-R intervals.

Causes of Premature Atrial Contraction

A number of conditions can cause a premature atrial contraction, such as an enlarged atrium. In an enlarged atrium, the myocardium is stretched, which disrupts the conduction pathways of the SA node impulses.

- **Left Atrium Enlargement:** This can be caused by left ventricle hypertrophy (enlarged left ventricle) or mitral stenosis (narrowing of the mitral valve).
- **Right Atrium Enlargement:** This can be caused by pulmonary hypertension (abnormally high blood pressure in arteries that supply the lungs) or tricuspid stenosis (narrowing of the tricuspid valve).

Other causes of premature atrial contraction are:

- Hypoxia (low oxygenated blood)
- Stress
- Caffeine
- Nicotine
- Myocardial ischemia (reduced blood supply to the heart)
- Sympathomimetic medications (mimetic the sympathetic nervous system's ability to increase the heart rate) such as epinephrine and norepinephrine

Treatment of Premature Atrial Contraction

Premature atrial contraction is treated by addressing the underlying cause. This includes:

- Administering supplemental oxygen
- Rest and relaxation
- Eliminating caffeine or nicotine
- Administering antianginal medication to increase blood flow to the heart
- Reducing the dose or eliminate sympathomimetic medications

Nonconducted Premature Atrial Contraction

A nonconducted premature atrial contraction (Figure 7.6) occurs when the ectopic atrial pacemaker's impulse is not conducted by the AV node to the ventricles because the AV node has not been repolarized.

It is easy to mis identify the nonconducted premature atrial contraction on an ECG because the nonconducted premature atrial contraction appears as a P wave without a QRS complex, which is similar to the wave pattern of a cardiac block, such as a Mobitz 1 or Wenckebach.

The nonconducted premature atrial contraction is distinguishable on an ECG by a distorted T wave preceding the pause caused by the premature atrial contraction. The cause and treatment of a nonconducted premature atrial contraction is the same as that of a premature atrial contraction.

7.4   Atrial Escape Beat

An atrial escape beat is a protective mechanism that maintains the heart rate. An atrial escape beat occurs when the SA node impulse is slowed or suppressed, such as in an atrial pause or cardiac arrest, or if the SA node impulse is blocked from depolarizing the ventricles (Figure 7.7). This has similar morphology to a premature atrial contraction except the impulse arrives later in the cardiac cycle.

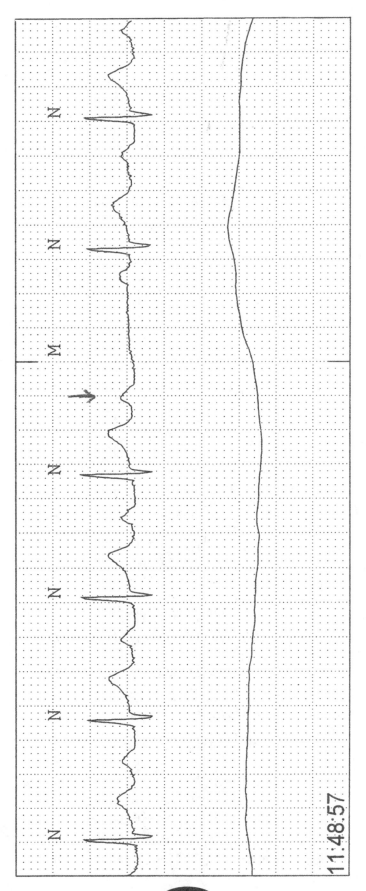

Figure 7.6 Nonconducted PAC.

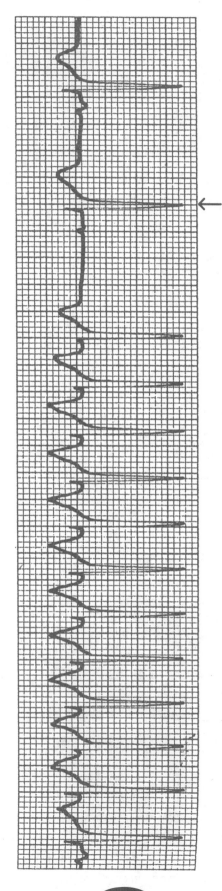

Figure 7.7 Burst of SVT, followed by an atrial escape beat. Notice how different the P wave looks.

The atrial escape beat appears on the ECG like a PAC except that the atrial escape beat comes late in the cycle. The escape beat is caused by the backup pacemaker site in the heart. There is no treatment for an atrial escape beat because this is a safety net that provides a backup pacemaker to the heart.

7.5 Wandering Atrial Pacemaker (WAP)

A wandering atrial pacemaker (Figure 7.8) is a normal phenomenon during sleep and in athletes in whom the vagal tone is naturally stimulated, causing the SA node to decrease its firing rate but stay within the normal 60 to 100 rates per minute. As a result, an ectopic atrial pacemaker's impulses take over.

The SA node's firing rate returns to normal as the vagal tone subsides, enabling the SA node to return to its role and decreasing the effect of the ectopic atrial pacemaker. The vagal tone is an impulse from the vagus nerve that decreases the SA node's firing rate, normally resulting in a decreased heart rate.

A wandering atrial pacemaker is not clinically significant because patients are usually asymptomatic. If the heart rate drops and the patient become symptomatic, vagal tone can be decreased by coughing, which returns the patient to a normal heart rate.

There is not one set of conditions that cause a wandering atrial pacemaker. However, patients who are predisposed to a wandering atrial pacemaker are those with:

- **Multifocal Atrial Tachycardia (MAT):** This is a heart rate >100 bpm caused by an atrial pacemaker. If the heart rate falls to ≤100 bpm, it becomes a wandering atrial pacemaker.

- **Chronic Obstructive Pulmonary Disease (COPD):** COPD patients have increased vagal tone.

Wandering Atrial Pacemaker and the ECG

The wandering atrial pacemaker is depicted on an ECG as changes in the P wave as the pacemaker wanders around the atria. The PR interval may vary depending on the ectopic site's proximity to the AV node.

7.6 Paroxysmal Atrial Tachycardia (PAT)

Paroxysmal atrial tachycardia, also known as a supraventricular tachycardia (SVT), is a sudden increase in heart rate between 140 and 250 bpm that suddenly returns to a normal heart rate of 60 to 100 bpm. An irritable ectopic atrial pacemaker that is usually initiated with more than three consecutive premature atrial contractions causes this.

Paroxysmal atrial tachycardia can occur with patients who have healthy or diseased hearts. Some patients may tolerate paroxysmal atrial tachycardia, whereas other patients may experience palpitations.

In paroxysmal atrial tachycardia there is less time spent in the heart filled with blood (diastole). Cardiac oxygen consumption increases, generating signs of angina (dyspnea and chest pain). The patient may show signs of altered mental status, anxiety, and shortness of breath.

Paroxysmal Atrial Tachycardia and the ECG

Paroxysmal atrial tachycardia (Figure 7.9) has the following characteristics on an ECG:

- **P Wave:** This is difficult to assess because the P wave is hidden by the T wave. When cardiac rhythm slows, there is one P wave for every QRS complex unless there is an underlying AV block.

- **PR Interval:** This is not measurable because of distortion of the P wave.

WAP→ wandering atrial pacemaker
variations in 'p' structure
3 different morphologies in 'p' structure

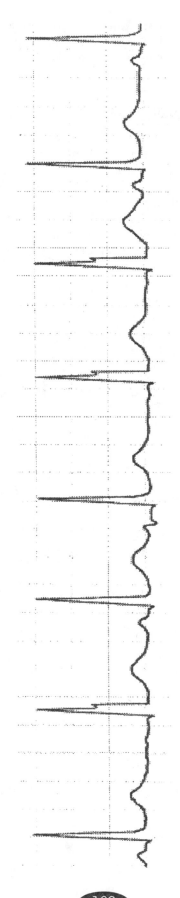

Figure 7.8 Wandering atrial pacemaker.

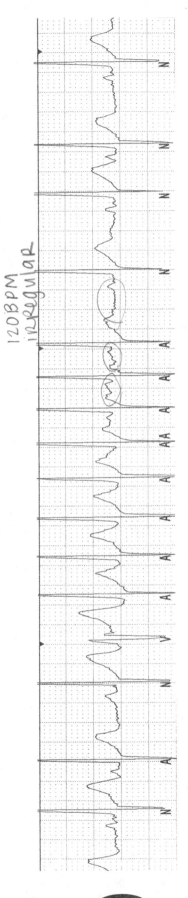

120BPM
irregular

SVT

Figure 7.9 Paroxysmal atrial tachycardia.

P waves hidden by T waves

Supraventricular tachycardia

103

Causes of Paroxysmal Atrial Tachycardia

A number of conditions can cause a paroxysmal atrial tachycardia. These are:

- **Atrial Automaticity:** Increases in the atrial pacemaker activity can result in increased cardiac rhythm.
- **Intra-atrial Re-entry:** In a normal cardiac cycle, impulses from the SA node terminate at the ventricles. However, impulses from the atrial pacemaker circulate within the atria.
- Caffeine
- Stress
- Alcohol
- Drug toxicity (digoxin)
- Chronic obstructive pulmonary disease (COPD)
- Pericarditis (inflamed pericardium)

Treatment of Paroxysmal Atrial Tachycardia

Paroxysmal atrial tachycardia is treated by:

- Using Valsalva's maneuver (forcible exhalation against a closed airway) if the patient is hemodynamically stable.
  - Have the patient close his or her mouth.
  - Pinch the nose closed.
  - Forcibly exhale.
- Administer adenosine (Adenocard) (see Chapter 12), if there is an acute onset.
- Administer antiarrhythmic medication (quinidine, procainamide, Rythmol, Ethmozine, amiodarone, sotalol, Tikosyn, or covert).
- Radiofrequency Ablation: This is an invasive procedure that uses electrodes to generate heat that destroys the tissues that are acting as the atrial pacemaker.
- Synchronized cardioversion (see Chapter 12) is used if the patient has a systolic blood pressure <90, is short of breath, and has altered mental status.

7.7   Atrial Flutter

Impulses from the atrial ectopic pacemaker follow a circular pathway from the right atrium to the left atrium then back to the right atrium, forming a re-entry circuit. These impulses cause rapid polarization and repolarization of the atrials at a rate of 250 to 300 bpm, resulting in a flutter called *atrial flutter*.

The AV node usually conducts half the SA impulse. This causes the loss of the atrial kick, causing decreased filling. The heart rate may increase to meet metabolic demands or the ventricular response may be 125 to 150. As a result, the patient may experience:

- Poor exercise tolerance
- Mild dyspnea
- Palpitations

Atrial Flutter and the ECG

Atrial flutter (Figure 7.10) has the following characteristics on an ECG:

- **P Wave:** The P wave initially shows a negative deflection followed by a positive deflection, creating a saw tooth appearance or the teeth of a hand saw found between the QRS complexes, called *flutter waves.*
- **QRS Complex:** The QRS complex size is <0.10 (normal). The ratio of QRS complex to P waves represents the conduction ratio (the number of SA impulses conducted by the AV node).
  - *3:1 Conduction Ratio:* One QRS complex for every three P waves.
  - *2:1 Conduction Ratio:* One QRS complex for every two P waves.
  - *Variable Conduction:* Variable atrial flutter has variable conduction ratios; therefore, the patient has an irregular heart rate.
- **PR Interval:** The PR interval cannot be measured because of the fast rate of the atrium.

Causes of Atrial Flutter

A number of conditions can cause atrial flutter. These are:

- **Hyperthyroidism:** Hypermetabolic state caused by increased T3 and T4.
- **Longstanding Hypertension:** Chronic high blood pressure.
- **Valvular Heart Disease:** The mitral, aortic, pulmonary, or tricuspid valves are diseased.
- **Chronic Obstructive Pulmonary Disease (COPD):** Chronic pulmonary disease.
- **Pericarditis (inflamed pericardium):** The outer lining of the heart is inflamed.
- **Heart Failure:** The heart is not pumping effectively.
- **Pulmonary Embolism:** A blood clot in the pulmonary vessels.

Treatment of Atrial Flutter

How to treat atrial flutter:

- **Control the Ventricular Rate:** Administer drugs known as calcium channel blockers (Cardizem, verapamil) or beta-adrenergic blockers (Lopressor).
  - *Caution:* These medications may cause acute exacerbation of heart failure in patients who have impaired left ventricular function.
- **Mechanism of Action:** Mechanism of action of calcium channel blockers and beta blockers:
  - *Calcium Channel Blockers:* Block the movement of calcium into the cells, thus causing a decrease in heart activity
  - *Beta Blockers:* Block The body's response to the naturally occurring catecholamines called epinephrine and norepinephrine, causing decreased excitation of the heart
- **Anticoagulants:** The patient is also at risk for embolization (clot) if the atrial flutter is present for more than 48 hours. Administer anticoagulants to prevent embolization.
- **Cardioversion:** Synchronized cardioversion at 100J is performed if the patient is hemodynamically unstable (hypotension and poor perfusion).

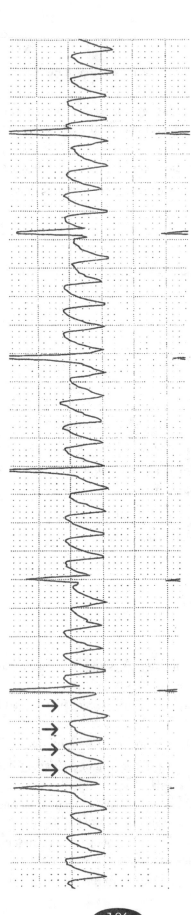

Figure 7.10 Atrial flutter with a 4:1 conduction.

4 p waves : 1 QRS complex

- ○ Oral anticoagulants are administered for three weeks before cardioversion and four weeks after cardioversion.

- ○ IV heparin is administered for 24 hours, then a transesophageal echocardiogram is performed, a procedure in which an ultrasound wand is inserted into the esophagus after the patient is sedated to assess heart function and detect any clots in the atrium. If there are no clots, then cardioversion is performed followed by administration of anticoagulation for four weeks.

- **Administer Adenosine:** This may slow the cardiac rhythm to reveal flutter waves. If the rhythm is revealed to be an A-flutter, adenosine is not the treatment of choice.

- **Radiofrequency Ablation:** This is an invasive procedure that uses electrodes to generate heat, which destroys the tissues that are acting as the atrial pacemaker.

7.8 Atrial Fibrillation

Atrial fibrillation causes the atrials to quiver at a rate in excess of 400 bpm, preventing the atrial kick from occurring. The atrials lose efficient pumping capability, resulting in diminished cardiac output and poor perfusion.

The ventricles' increased depolarization and repolarization rate causes increased oxygen consumption and decreased filling time. The loss of the atrial kick causes a reduction up to 30% of the stroke volume, which has a negative effect on patients who have underlying heart disease or low cardiac ejection fraction.

The patient may experience:

- Low blood pressure

- Exercise intolerance

- Chest pain

- Mild to moderate shortness of breath

Blood pools in the atrial chambers, presenting an opportunity for mural thrombi (clot) to form. This places the patient at risk for a pulmonary embolism (clot in the right atrium), stroke, or arterial occlusion of the extremities, intestines, or kidneys.

Atrial Fibrillation and the ECG

Atrial fibrillation has the following characteristics on an ECG:

- **P Wave:** The P wave is not discernible.

- **PR Interval:** The PR interval cannot be measured.

- **QRS Complex:** The QRS complex is narrowed. The size of the QRS complex depends on if the AV node can control the ventricular response.

- ○ *Controlled Impulse:* The QRS complex is <100.

- ○ *Uncontrolled Impulse:* The QRS complex is ≥100.

- **Wave Form:** Quivering produces a fine or coarse fibrillatory wave, or a combination of both, which is referred to as fib-flutter.

- **Heart Rate:** Irregular.

- Rates of 100 bpm are called controlled atrial fibrillation (Figure 7.11).
- Rates >100 bpm are called uncontrolled atrial fibrillation or rapid atrial fibrillation (Figure 7.12).

Causes of Atrial Fibrillation

A number of conditions can cause atrial fibrillation:

- Pulmonary hypertension
- Left ventricle dysfunction
- Mitral/tricuspid valve disease (most common cause)
- Stress
- Cocaine, methamphetamines, or stimulants
- Excessive alcohol intake (holiday heart syndrome)
- Coronary heart disease
- Diabetes
- Hyperthyroidism
- Cardiomyopathy
- Postcardiac revascularization—bypass surgery

Treatment of Atrial Fibrillation

The treatment of atrial fibrillation depends on whether this is a new onset that occurs <48 hours or chronic atrial fibrillation.

- **New Onset:**
  - The patient is hemodynamically unstable:
    - Perform synchronized cardioversion and admit the patient to the hospital.
  - The patient is hemodynamically stable:
    - If the patient's INR is 2 to 3 for three weeks, do one of the following:
      - Perform synchronized cardioversion.
      - Administer calcium channel blocker (diltiazem).
      - Administer beta blocker (metoprolol).
      - Follow up on an outpatient basis in 24 to 48 hours.
    - If the patient's INR is <2.0 or the patient is not on anticoagulants, perform a transesophageal echocardiogram to detect any atrial clots.
      - If no clots are discovered, employ synchronized cardioversion.
      - Follow up on an outpatient basis in 24 to 48 hours.
- **Chronic Atrial Fibrillation:**
  - Perform cardiac rhythm control:
    - Treat the underlying cause.

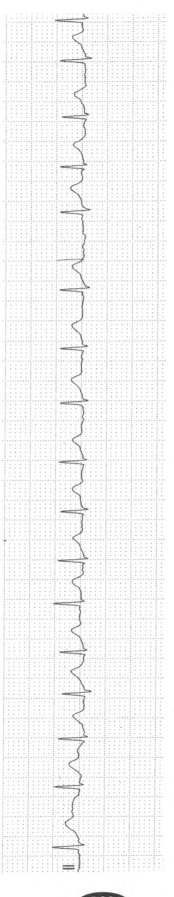

Figure 7.11 Uncontrolled atrial fibrillation.

120 bpm
undescernable p wave
Uncontr. atrial fibrillation ectopic foci in atria

109

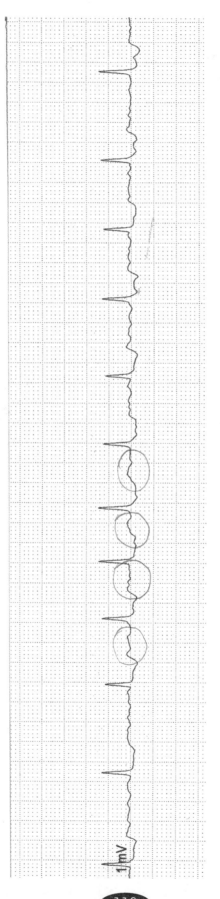

Figure 7.12 Controlled atrial fibrillation.

90 bpm
Irregular Rhythm
P interval undiscernable
Controlled atrial fibrillation

- ▪ Administer amiodarone.

- ▪ Administer antiarrhythmic (sotalol) and monitor the ECG for a prolonged QT interval and monitor electrolytes.

  ○ Treat the symptoms of atrial fibrillation.

  ○ Maintain ventricular rate control if the patient has a cardiac rate of 60 to 80 bpm at rest or 100 to 115 beats after moderate exercise.

  - ▪ Block the AV node by administering a beta blocker, calcium channel blocker, or digoxin. Both beta blockers and calcium channel blockers can be given together if single-dose therapy fails.

  - ▪ Administer antiarrhythmic medication (amiodarone).

  - ▪ Radiofrequency Ablation: This is an invasive procedure that uses electrodes to generate heat that destroys the tissues that are acting as the atrial pacemaker.

  ○ Administer anticoagulates (warfarin) to prevent clots and strokes.

Solved Problems

Ectopic Pacemaker

7.1   What is enhanced/suppressed automaticity?

Enhanced/suppressed automaticity occurs when the cardiac cells in the ectopic pacemaker fire at a faster rate than the rate of the SA node. As a result, the SA node's automaticity (ability to automatically generate an impulse) is suppressed as the SA node relinquishes control of the ectopic pacemaker.

7.2   What is triggered activity?

Triggered activity (after depolarization) occurs when the ectopic pacemaker is triggered to fire an impulse after depolarization and before repolarization, resulting in couplets (two beats) or triplets (three beats) per cardiac cycle.

7.3   What causes the triggered activity?

Prolonged QT intervals, bradycardias, hypomagnesemia, hypoxia, and digoxin toxicity cause triggered activity.

7.4   What is re-entry?

In a normal cardiac cycle, the impulse travels from the SA node in the atria and ends in the ventricles. In re-entry, the impulse travels in a circular path returning to the SA node. The impulse continues as long as there is a refractory period within the circle of conduction. A refractory period is the amount of time it takes for an excitable membrane to be ready for a second stimulus once it returns to its resting state after excitation. Re-entry is responsible for most atrial flutters (abnormal heart rhythm in the atrium), paroxysmal atrial tachycardia (a regular, fast heartbeat starting in the atria that begins and ends, suddenly), and some ventricular tachycardias (a regular, fast heart rate originating in the ventricles).

Atrial Arrhythmias

7.5   What is atrial fibrillation?

Atrial fibrillation is the most common arrhythmia involving the atria. Normal impulses generated by the SA node become suppressed by impulses generated by an ectopic pacemaker located in the atria, resulting in the quivering (fibrillating) of the atrial cardiac muscle rather than coordinated contractions.

7.6   What is atrial flutter?

Atrial flutter is an arrhythmia caused by a re-entry rhythm of either the right or left atrium, which is caused by an ectopic pacemaker that generates a premature impulse, resulting in a self-perpetuating loop as the premature impulse moves through atrial cardiac muscle. As a result, the patient feels regular heart palpitations.

Premature Atrial Contraction

7.7   What is a premature atrial contraction?

A premature atrial contraction is an impulse before the SA node impulse that originates from one or more atrial ectopic pacemakers that disrupts the normal sinus rhythm. Once the premature impulse reaches the AV node, the conduction path of the impulse follows the same path as the SA node impulse.

7.8   What might frequent premature atrial contractions indicate?

Frequent premature atrial contractions might indicate that the atria are being irritated, which could lead to atrial fibrillation or atrial flutter.

7.9   What is a quadrigeminal premature atrial contraction?

A quadrigeminal premature atrial contraction occurs when there is a premature atrial contraction every fourth beat.

7.10   What is premature atrial tachycardia?

Premature atrial tachycardia (PAT) is more than three series of premature atrial contractions, which implies that sudden starts and breaks occur in the atrial ectopic pacemaker.

7.11   How are premature atrial contractions depicted on an ECG?

Premature atrial contractions are depicted on an ECG as abnormal P waves that may be hidden in the preceding T wave, in which case the T wave is distorted. The ECG shows aberrantly conducted PCAs, which are wide or notched QRS complexes.

A premature atrial contraction might be difficult to detect on an ECG because the impulse from the ectopic pacemaker follows the same conduction path as the SA node impulse. That is, the QRS complex is the same as that of the SA node impulse.

Adding a further complication, it is confusing to differentiate between premature atrial contractions and premature ventricular contractions. The best way to make the distinction on the ECG is to identify an abnormal P wave and a distorted T wave.

7.12   What is a noncompensatory pause?

A noncompensatory pause occurs when early depolarization of the atria resets the timing of the SA node. The measurement of the pause is less than two R-R intervals in the underlying regular rhythm.

7.13   What is a compensatory pause?

A compensatory pause occurs when SA-node timing is not reset by the PAC. The measurement of the pause is equal to two R-R intervals in the underlying regular rhythm.

7.14   What can cause premature atrial contractions?

Left atrium enlargement, right atrium enlargement, hypoxia (low-oxygenated blood), stress, caffeine, nicotine, myocardial ischemia (reduced blood supply to the heart), and sympathomimetic medications (mimic the sympathetic nervous system's ability to increase the heart rate) such as epinephrine and norepinephrine can cause premature atrial contractions. Left atrial enlargement can be caused by left ventrical hypertrophy (enlarged left ventricle) or mitral stenosis (narrowing of the mitral valve). Right atrial enlargement can be caused by pulmonary hypertension (abnormally high blood pressure in arteries that supply the lungs) or tricuspid stenosis (narrowing of the tricuspid valve).

7.15   How is premature atrial contraction treated?

Premature atrial contraction is treated by addressing the underlying cause, which may include administering supplemental oxygen, prescribing rest and relaxation, eliminating caffeine or nicotine, administering antianginal medication to increase blood flow to the heart, and reducing the dose or eliminating sympathomimetic medications.

7.16   What is a nonconducted premature atrial contraction?

A nonconducted premature atrial contraction occurs when the ectopic atrial pacemaker's impulse is not conducted by the AV node to the ventricles because the AV node has not repolarized.

Atrial Escape Beat

7.17   What is an atrial escape beat?

An atrial escape beat is a protective mechanism that maintains the heart rate. An atrial escape beat occurs when the SA node impulse is slowed or suppressed such as in an atrial pause or cardiac arrest, or if the SA node impulse is blocked from depolarizing the ventricles. This has similar morphology to a premature atrial contraction except the impulse arrives later in the cardiac cycle.

Wandering Atrial Pacemaker

7.18   What is a wandering atrial pacemaker?

A wandering atrial pacemaker is a normal phenomenon during sleep and in athletes in whom the vagal tone is naturally stimulated, causing the SA node to decrease its firing rate but stay within the normal 60 to 100 bpm. As a result, an ectopic atrial pacemaker's impulses take over.

7.19   What is a multifocal atrial tachycardia?

Multifocal atrial tachycardia (MAT) is a heart rate >100 bpm caused by an atrial pacemaker. If the heart rate falls to 100 bpm or less, it becomes a wandering atrial pacemaker.

7.20   How does a wandering atrial pacemaker present on an ECG?

The wandering atrial pacemaker is depicted on an ECG as changes in the P wave as the pacemaker wanders around the atria. The PR interval may also vary with a shorter PR interval, occurring the closer the pacemaker site is to the AV node.

Paroxysmal Atrial Tachycardia

7.21   What is paroxysmal atrial tachycardia?

Paroxysmal atrial tachycardia, also known as a supraventricular tachycardia (SVT), is a sudden increase in heart rate between 140 and 250 bpm that suddenly returns to a normal heart rate of 60 to 100 bpm.

7.22   What causes paroxysmal atrial tachycardia?

This is caused by an irritable ectopic atrial pacemaker that is usually initiated with more than three consecutive premature atrial contractions.

7.23   Why might a patient who has paroxysmal atrial tachycardia show signs of altered mental status?

In paroxysmal atrial tachycardia there is less time spent as the heart fills with blood (diastole). Cardiac oxygen consumption increases, generating signs of angina (dyspnea and chest pain). The patient may show signs of altered mental status, anxiety, and shortness of breath.

7.24   How does paroxysmal atrial tachycardia appear on an ECG?

Paroxysmal atrial tachycardia has the following characteristics on an ECG:

- **P Wave:** This is difficult to assess because the P wave is hidden by the T wave. When the cardiac rhythm slows, there is one P wave for every QRS complex unless there is an underlying AV block.

- **PR Interval:** The PR interval is not measurable because of P wave distortion.

7.25   What might cause paroxysmal atrial tachycardia?

Several conditions can cause paroxysmal atrial tachycardia:

- Atrial Automaticity: Increases in the atrial pacemaker activity can result in increased cardiac rhythm.

- Intra-atrial Re-entry: In a normal cardiac cycle, impulses from the SA node terminate at the ventricles. However, impulses from the atrial pacemaker circulate within the atrials.

- Caffeine

- Stress

- Alcohol

- Drug toxicity (digoxin)

- Chronic obstructive pulmonary disease (COPD)

- Pericarditis (inflamed pericardium)

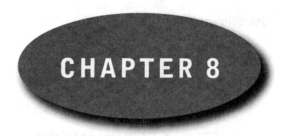

Junctional Rhythms

8.1 Definition

The cardiac rate is determined by the SA node, which is called the heart's pacemaker. Impulses from the SA node sinus rhythm depolarize the atria and pass from the atria through the bundle of His, the bundle branches, and then along the Purkinje fiber to the ventricles.

If conduction of impulses from the SA node is slowed or blocked, the ectopic pacemaker near the AV node takes over as the heart's pacemaker, resulting in a junctional rhythm. The atria may contract before, during, or after the ventricles contract; however, this occurs using a pathway that is alternative to the SA node pathway.

- **Junctional Beat:** Less than three impulses generated by the AV node or the AV junction
- **Junctional Rhythm:** Three or more impulses generated by the AV node or the AV junction

Common junctional rhythms are:

- Junctional escape beat
- Accelerated junctional
- Junctional tachycardia
- Premature junctional contraction

8.2 Junctional Rhythms and Retrograde Conduction

A junctional rhythm begins either by an ectopic pacemaker located at the AV node or in the AV junction when the rate of impulses from the SA node falls below the rate of the AV node. When the impulse originates in junctional tissue, the atrial depolarization is retrograde. Retrograde is when the impulse flows backward through the atria.

Junctional Rhythms and ECG

The P wave will be negative in lead II because there is retrograde depolarization of the atria (Figure 8.1). The ectopic pacemaker site closest to the AV node dictates the characteristics of the P wave.

- **Atrial Depolarization Occurs First:** The P wave comes before the QRS complex.
- **Atria and Ventricles are Depolarized Simultaneously:** The P wave is buried in the QRS complex.
- **Atrial Depolarization Occurs After Ventricular Depolarization:** The P wave is after the QRS complex.

The ECG will also show:

- **PR Interval:** <0.10 seconds because the impulse from the ectopic pacemaker site is close to the AV node
- **QRS Complex:** Narrow because ventricles are depolarized through the normal conduction pathways

8.3   Junctional Escape Rhythm

A junctional escape rhythm (Figure 8.2) occurs when the SA node is suppressed to a level where the ectopic pacemaker at the AV junction takes over as the primary cardiac pacemaker. This may also occur when the impulse from the SA node does not reach the AV junction within 1.5 seconds.

Junctional Escape Rhythm and ECG

A junctional escape rhythm has the following ECG characteristics:

- **P Wave:** Inverted in lead II. P wave occurs before or after the QRS complex or the P wave may not be present.
- **PR Interval:** <0.10 seconds.
- **Heart Rate:** Between 40 and 60 bpm.
- **Rhythm:** Regular if there is an escape beat; irregular if there is an escape rhythm.

Causes of a Junctional Escape Rhythm

Common causes of a junctional escape rhythm are:

- **Sick Sinus Syndrome:** Malfunction of the SA node.
- **Digoxin Toxicity:** Caused by conduction depression.
- **Ischemia of the AV Node:** Especially with acute inferior infarction involving the posterior descending artery, which is the origin of the AV nodal artery branch.
- **Post–Cardiac Surgery:** Caused by inflammation.

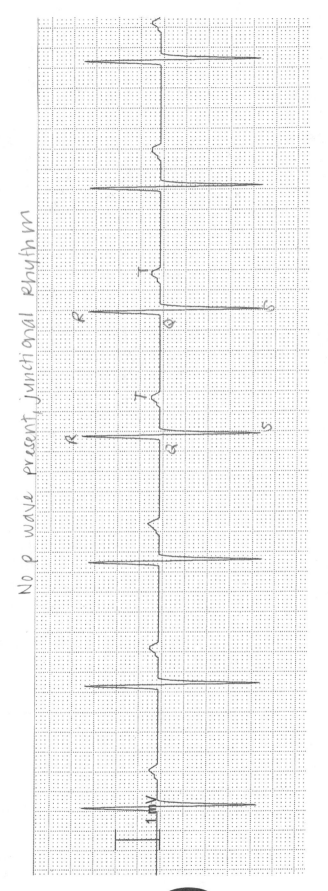

Figure 8.1 Junctional rhythm rate of 50.

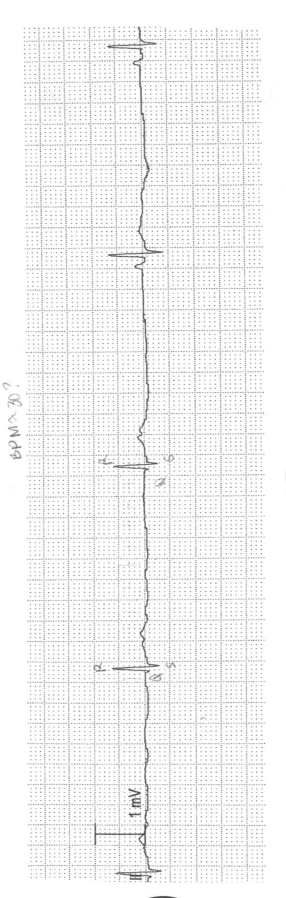

Figure 8.2 Junctional escape converting to a sinus bradycardia.

- **Acute Inflammation (i.e., acute rheumatic fever, Lyme disease):** Inflammation involves the conduction system. The conduction system is sensitive to inflammation.

- **Medication That Causes Sinus Bradycardia (i.e., beta blockers, calcium blockers, antiarrhythmic agents):** The medication slows impulse generation by the SA node below the threshold when the AV node naturally takes over as the primary cardiac pacemaker.

- **Isoproterenol Infusion.**

- **Metabolic States That Increase Adrenergic Tone.**

Treatment of a Junctional Escape Rhythm

The treatment of junctional escape rhythm depends on whether the patient is symptomatic and on the underlying cause.

- If the junctional escape rhythm is the result of increased vagal tone and the patient is asymptomatic, then no treatment is warranted.

- If the junctional escape rhythm results in the loss of atrial kick leading to decreased cardiac function, then increase the cardiac output by temporary pacing and treat the underlying cause of the junctional escape rhythm.

- If the junctional escape rhythm is the result of sick sinus syndrome or AV block(s), then the patient requires insertion of a permanent pacemaker.

- If the junctional escape rhythm is the result of digoxin toxicity, then administer digoxin immune Fab (Digibind).

8.4   Premature Junctional Contraction (PJC)

Premature junctional contraction is an impulse from the ectopic pacemaker site in the AV junction that occurs early in the cardiac cycle.

ECG characteristics of a premature junctional contraction are:

- **P Wave:** Inverted in lead II. P wave occurs just before or after the QRS complex or is not present at all.
- **PR Interval:** <0.10 seconds
- **QRS Complex:** Appears premature but normal
- **Rhythm:**
  - *Couplets:* Two sequential premature junctional contractions
  - *Triplets:* Three sequential premature junctional contractions
  - *Junctional Rhythm:* More than three sequential premature junctional contractions
- Distinguish from a premature atrial contraction
  - Premature atrial contraction is more common than a premature junctional contraction
  - *P Wave:* Consider the premature junctional contraction if the P wave is:
    - Not obvious
    - Inverted
    - After the QRS

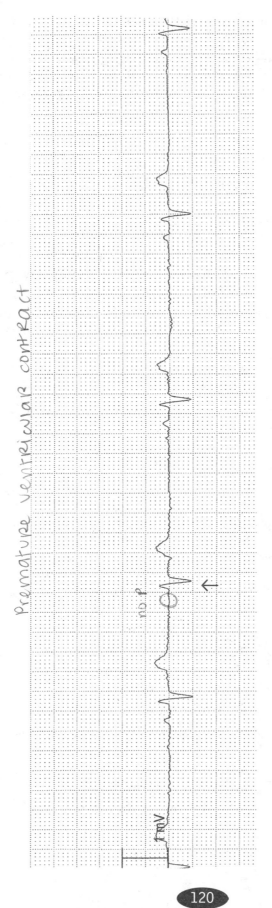

Figure 8.3 Premature junctional escape.

Causes and Treatment of Premature Junctional Contraction

Common causes of premature junctional contraction are:

- Digitalis toxicity
- Enhanced automaticity of the AV node
- Coronary artery disease (CAD)
- Heart failure
- Valve disease
- Irritated myocardium from hypoxemia

No treatment is necessary for premature junctional contraction. Frequent premature junctional contractions are a sign that the patient may be developing a junctional rhythm.

8.5   Accelerated Junctional Rhythm

An accelerated junctional rhythm (Figure 8.4) is similar to a junctional escape rhythm except the cardiac rate is between 60 and 100 bpm. A junctional escape rhythm has a cardiac rate of between 40 and 60 bpm.
    The ECG characteristics are:

- **P Wave:** Inverted in lead II. P wave occurs before or after the QRS complex or the P wave may not be present.
- **PR Interval:** <0.10 seconds.
- **Heart Rate:** Between 40 and 60 bpm.
- **Rhythm:** Regular.

Common Causes of Accelerated Junctional Rhythm

Common causes of an accelerated junctional rhythm are:

- **Digoxin Toxicity:** The slowing of conduction through the AV node may be substantial enough that the AV tissue may assume the role of the pacemaker.
- **Ischemia of the AV Node:** Especially with acute inferior infarction involving the posterior descending artery, which is the origin of the AV nodal artery branch.
- **Post–Cardiac Surgery:** Inflammation affecting the conduction pathways.
- **Acute Inflammation (i.e. acute rheumatic fever, Lyme disease):** The inflammation involves the conduction system.
- **Medication That Causes Sinus Bradycardia (i.e., beta blockers, calcium blockers, antiarrhythmic agents):** The medication slows impulse generation by the SA node below the threshold when the AV node naturally takes over as the primary cardiac pacemaker.
- **Isoproterenol Infusion.**

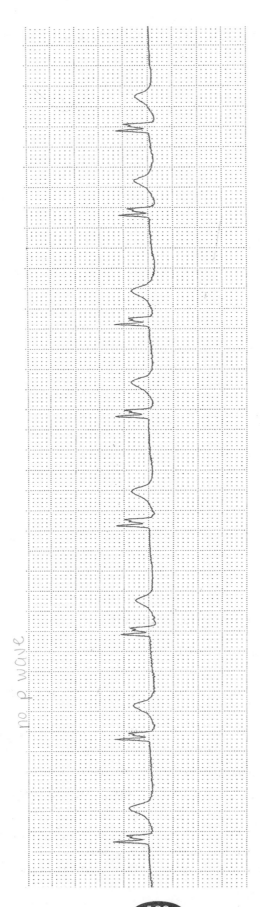

no p wave

Figure 8.4 Accelerated junctional rhythm.

- **Anoxia or Acidosis:** Increases the adrenergic tone or makes it less likely to respond to catecholamines such as norepinephrine.

- **Heart Failure.**

Treatment of an Accelerated Junctional Rhythm

The treatment of an accelerated junctional rhythm depends on whether the patient is symptomatic and on the underlying cause.

- No treatment is necessary if the cardiac rate of the accelerated junctional rhythm is the same as the rate of impulses from the SA node. There is adequate perfusion and the patient is asymptomatic.

- Review the patient's medications to determine if one or more medications might be the cause of accelerated junctional rhythm.

- Assess if the patient's decreased cardiac function is caused by the loss of an atrial kick. A pacemaker may be indicated to restore AV synchronization and the atrial kick and treat the underlying cause, such as Digibind for digoxin toxicity.

- Administer digoxin immune Fab (Digibind) if the accelerated junctional rhythm is caused by digoxin toxicity.

8.6   Paroxysmal Junctional Tachycardia (PJT)

Paroxysmal junctional tachycardia (Figure 8.5) occurs when an ectopic pacemaker located near the AV junction becomes the primary cardiac pacemaker and sends impulses at a rate greater than 100 impulses per minute.
The ECG characteristics are:

- **P Wave:** Inverted in lead II. P wave occurs before or after the QRS complex or the P wave may not be present.

- **PR Interval:** <0.10 seconds.

- **Heart Rate:** >100 bpm.

- **Rhythm:** Regular.

- Distinguish between paroxysmal junctional tachycardia (PJT) and paroxysmal atrial tachycardia (PAT):

  ○ PAT more common than PJT.

  ○ If a definite determination cannot be made, then the patient has supraventricular tachycardia (SVT).

  ○ Administer adenosine to slow down the heart enough to differentiate a PJT from a PAT.

  ○ P Wave:

    ▪ PJT: Hidden in the QRS complex

    ▪ PAT: Hidden in preceding T wave

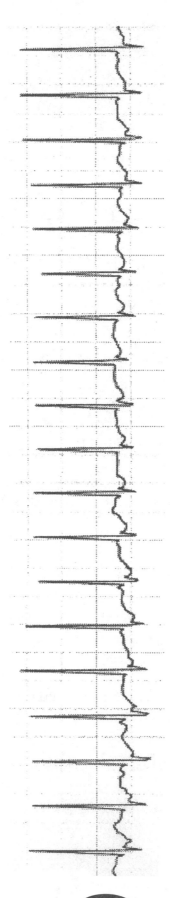

Figure 8.5 Junctional tachycardia.

Cause of Paroxysmal Junctional Tachycardia (PJT)

Common causes of a paroxysmal junctional tachycardia are:

- **Digoxin Toxicity:** The slowing of conduction through the AV node may be substantial enough that the AV tissue may assume the role of the pacemaker.

- **Ischemia of the AV Node:** Especially with acute inferior infarction involving the posterior descending artery, which is the origin of the AV nodal artery branch.

- **Post–Cardiac Surgery:** Inflammation or damage to the pathways.

- **Acute Inflammation (i.e., acute rheumatic fever, Lyme disease):** The conduction pathways are susceptible to inflammation that involves the conduction system.

- **Medication That Causes Sinus Bradycardia (i.e., beta blockers, calcium blockers, antiarrhythmic agents):** The medication slows impulse generation by the SA node below the threshold when the AV node naturally takes over as the primary cardiac pacemaker.

- **Heart Failure.**

Treatment of Paroxysmal Junctional Tachycardia (PJT)

The patient may decompensate quickly because the fast heart rate results in increased consumption of oxygen and the patient lost 30% of the cardiac stroke volume due to absence of the atrial kick.

The treatment of paroxysmal junctional tachycardia is:

1. Slow the heart rate while preserving cardiac output by administering diltiazem or a beta blocker.

2. Administer oxygen.

3. Correct the underlying cause.

Note that administration of adenosine and synchronized cardioversion is not effective.

Solved Problems

Junctional Rhythms

8.1 What is a junctional rhythm?

If conduction of impulses from the SA node is slowed or blocked, the ectopic pacemaker near the AV node takes over as the heart's pacemaker, resulting in a junctional rhythm. The atria contract before the ventricles; however, this occurs using a pathway that is alternative to the SA node pathway.

8.2 What is a junctional beat?

A junctional beat is less than three impulses generated by the AV node or the AV junction.

8.3 What are common junctional rhythms?

Common junctional rhythms are junctional escape beat, accelerated junctional, junctional tachycardia, and premature junctional contraction.

8.4 What is retrograde contraction?

Retrograde occurs when the impulse flows backward through the atria.

8.5 How does the P wave appear when atrial depolarization occurs first?

The P wave comes before the QRS complex.

8.6 How does the P wave appear when the atria and ventricles depolarize simultaneously?

The P wave is buried in the QRS complex.

8.7 How does the P wave appear when atrial depolarization occurs after ventricular depolarization?

The P wave occurs after the QRS complex.

8.8 Why is the PR interval <0.10 seconds in a junctional rhythm?

PR Interval is <0.10 seconds in a junctional rhythm because the impulse from the ectopic pacemaker site is close to the AV node.

Junctional Escape Rhythms

8.9 What is a junctional escape rhythm?

A junctional escape rhythm occurs when the SA node is suppressed to a level at which the ectopic pacemaker at the AV junction takes over as the primary cardiac pacemaker. This may also occur when the impulse from the SA node does not reach the AV junction within 1.5 seconds.

8.10 What are the ECG characteristics of a junctional escape rhythm?

- **P Wave:** Inverted in lead II. A P wave occurs before or after the QRS complex or the P wave may not be present.
- **PR Interval:** <0.10 seconds
- **Heart Rate:** Between 40 and 60 bpm
- **Rhythm:** It is regular if there is an escape beat, and irregular if there is an escape rhythm.

8.11 What are the causes of a junctional escape rhythm?

Causes of a junctional escape rhythm are sick sinus syndrome, structural heart defects, digoxin toxicity, ischemia of the AV node, post–cardiac surgery, acute inflammation, medication that causes sinus bradycardia, isoproterenol infusion, and metabolic states that increase adrenergic tone.

8.12 What is the treatment for a junctional escape rhythm that is caused by digoxin toxicity?

If the junctional escape rhythm is the result of digoxin toxicity, then administer digoxin immune Fab (Digibind).

8.13 What is the treatment for a junctional escape rhythm that is caused by sick sinus syndrome?

If the junctional escape rhythm is the result of sick sinus syndrome or AV block(s), then the patient requires insertion of a permanent pacemaker.

8.14   When might it be unwarranted to treat a junctional escape rhythm?

If the junctional escape rhythm is the result of increased vagal tone and the patient is asymptomatic, no treatment is warranted.

Premature Junctional Contraction

8.15   What is a premature junctional contraction?

A premature junctional contraction is an impulse from the ectopic pacemaker site in the AV junction that occurs early in the cardiac cycle.

8.16   How is a premature junctional contraction distinguished from a premature atrial contraction?

A premature atrial contraction is more common than a premature junctional contraction. Consider premature junctional contraction if the P wave is not obvious, is inverted, and occurs after the QRS.

8.17   What are causes of premature junctional contraction?

Common causes of premature junctional contraction are digitalis toxicity, enhanced automaticity of the AV node, CAD, heart failure, valve disease, and irritated myocardium from hypoxemia.

8.18   What is the treatment for premature junctional contraction?

No treatment is necessary for premature junctional contraction. Frequent premature junctional contractions are a sign that the patient may be developing a junctional rhythm.

Accelerated Junctional Rhythm

8.19   What is an accelerated junctional rhythm?

An accelerated junctional rhythm is similar to a junctional escape rhythm except the cardiac rate is 60 to 100 bpm. A junctional escape rhythm has a cardiac rate of 40 to 60 bpm.

8.20   What are causes of accelerated junctional rhythm?

Common causes of an accelerated junctional rhythm are digoxin toxicity, ischemia of the AV Node, post–cardiac surgery, acute inflammation, medication that causes sinus bradycardia, isoproterenol infusion, metabolic states that increase adrenergic tone, and heart failure.

8.21   What is the treatment for accelerated junctional rhythm?

- No treatment is necessary if the cardiac rate of the accelerated junctional rhythm is the same as the rate of impulses from the SA node. There is adequate perfusion and the patient is asymptomatic.

- Review the patient's medications to determine if one or more medications might be the cause of accelerated junctional rhythm.

- Assess if the patient's decreased cardiac function is cause by the loss of an atrial kick. If so, then increase the cardiac output by temporary atrial pacing and correcting volume status.

- Administer digoxin immune Fab (Digibind) if the accelerated junctional rhythm is caused by digoxin toxicity.

Paroxysmal Junctional Tachycardia

8.22   What is paroxysmal junctional tachycardia?

Paroxysmal junctional tachycardia occurs when an ectopic pacemaker located near the AV junction becomes the primary cardiac pacemaker and sends impulses at a rate greater than 100 impulses per minute.

8.23   What are the ECG characteristics of paroxysmal junctional tachycardia?

The ECG characteristics are:

- **P Wave:** Inverted in lead II. P wave occurs before or after the QRS complex or the P wave may not be present.

- **PR Interval:** <0.10 seconds

- **Heart Rate:** >100 bpm

- **Rhythm:** Regular

8.24   How does a health care provider distinguish between paroxysmal junctional tachycardia and paroxysmal atrial tachycardia?

A health care provider distinguishes between paroxysmal junctional tachycardia (PJT) and paroxysmal atrial tachycardia (PAT) by considering:

- That PAT is more common than PJT

- If a definite determine cannot be made, then the patient has supraventricular tachycardia (SVT)

- Administration of adenosine to slow down the heart enough to differentiate a PJT from a PAT.

- P Wave:

  o *PJT:* Hidden in the QRS complex

  o *PAT:* Hidden in preceding T wave

8.25   What might cause paroxysmal junctional tachycardia?

The conditions that might cause paroxysmal junctional tachycardia are digoxin toxicity, ischemia of the AV node, post–cardiac surgery, acute inflammation, medication that causes sinus bradycardia (i.e., beta blockers, calcium blockers, antiarrhythmic agents), theophylline or catecholamine infusion, and heart failure.

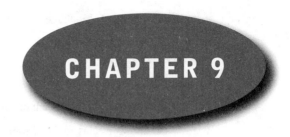

CHAPTER 9

Atrioventricular Blocks

9.1 Definition

A heart block is a disease of the conduction system of the heart, which can cause lightheadedness, fainting (syncope), and palpitations. Normal conduction of the cardiac impulse is initiated by the SA node and travels through the atria to the AV node. From the AV node, the cardiac impulse travels through the bundle of His, then to the bundle branches, and finally to the ventricles. In an AV heart block, the impulse is either delayed or terminated before the ventricles are depolarized.

9.2 AV Block and PR Interval

The distance between the P wave and the onset of the QRS complex on an ECG is the PR interval. The PR interval is the time the cardiac impulse takes to travel from the SA node to the point where the ventricles are depolarized. Ventricular depolarization occurs at the beginning of the QRS complex.

AV Block and Changes in the PR Interval

In a normal cardiac impulse, the PR interval is between 0.12 and 0.20 seconds. However, in an AV block, there is a noticeable change in the PR interval. These changes can be:

- A PR interval >0.20 seconds.
- Variation in the PR interval where the interval progressively becomes longer.
- No PR interval. There is no relationship between the P wave and the QRS complex.

9.3 Classification of AV Blocks

An AV block is the blockage of the cardiac impulse. AV blocks are classified in degrees at which the cardiac impulse is blocked. Over the patient's lifetime, an AV block can progress from the less harmful first-degree block to more threatening degrees.

There are three degrees of AV blockage:

- **First-Degree:** Less harmful
- **Second-Degree:** Divided into two types:
  - *Type 1:* Also known as Wenckebach or Mobitz 1
  - *Type 2:* Also known as classical or Mobitz 2
- **Third-Degree:** Complete heart block (CHB)

9.4 First-Degree AV Block

The first-degree AV block is the least life threatening (Figure 9.1). It is defined on the ECG as:

- **P Wave:** There is one P wave for every QRS complex.
- **PR Interval:** The P wave is delayed in the AV node longer than normal, resulting in a prolonged PR interval >0.20.
- **QRS Complex:** The QRS complex is normal because every P wave is conducted through to the ventricles.

Causes of a First-Degree AV Block

A first-degree AV block might occur in a healthy person when there is increased vagal tone, which means that increased impulses along the vagus nerve reduce cardiac impulses. Once stimulation to the vagus nerve stops, normal cardiac impulses return.

A first-degree AV block can also occur in a myocardial ischemia or infarct in the inferior wall of the heart. The right coronary artery supplies 90% of the blood to the AV node. Likewise, the circumflex artery supplies the AV node with 10% of its blood supply. If either or both of these arteries narrows, blood supply to the AV node decreases, therefore reducing the AV node cardiac impulse.

Other causes of a first-degree AV block are:

- **Endocarditis and Lyme Disease:** These diseases infect cardiac conduction pathways.
- **Medication:** Digitalis, beta blockers, calcium channel blockers, and amiodarone all slow cardiac conduction.
- **Age:** The cardiac conduction system degenerates with age.
- **Hyperkalemia:** Abnormally high levels of potassium can decrease cardiac conductivity.

Treatment of a First-Degree AV Block

A first-degree AV block is usually asymptomatic. The patient likely does not realize there is decreased AV node conductivity. Therefore, there is no treatment required for first-degree AV block.

However, the health care provider may monitor a patient's cardiac conductivity if the patient is administered medication that may affect cardiac conductivity. If it is found that the medication is causing a first-degree AV block, the health care provider may change or discontinue the medication, thereby restoring normal cardiac conductivity.

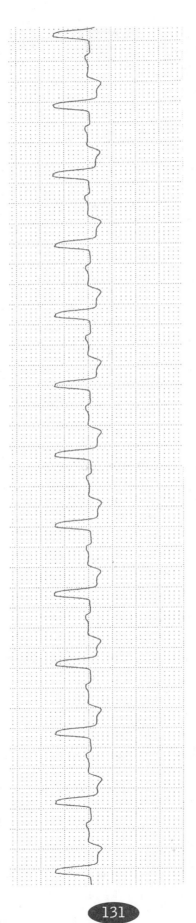

1st degree heart
block
PR greater
than 1 lg
box

Figure 9.1 NSR with a first-degree AV block, PR interval 0.24 seconds.

If a health care provider identifies a first-degree AV block during a routine examination, the health care provider is likely to monitor the patient's cardiac conductivity regularly because a first-degree AV block may progress to more symptomatic AV blocks.

9.5 Second-Degree AV Block Type 1

The second-degree type 1 AV block is referred to as Wenckebach or Mobitz 1 and is nearly always caused by a disease of the AV node. This type of AV block is seldom serious; however, it can progress into more serious AV block. The patient may report feeling an irregular heartbeat.

The atrial rhythm is regular and the ventricular rhythm is irregular. It is defined on the ECG as:

- **P Wave:** Some P waves are not followed by a QRS complex.

- **P-to-P Interval:** Distance between P waves is regular or the P-to-P interval maps out.

- **PR Interval:** The PR interval progressively lengthens because the impulse is held increasingly longer at the AV node until one impulse is not conducted through to the ventricles. This causes a nonconducted P wave, resulting in a pause that causes an atrial, junctional, or ventricular escape beat during the pause. Once the cardiac cycle is completed (lengthening of the PR interval and dropped beat), the cardiac cycle starts over. This is represented by a group of beats on the ECG.

- **QRS Complex:** The QRS complex represents cardiac impulses that are conducted through the AV node and will be <0.10 seconds on the ECG.

Second-Degree AV Block Type 1 vs. Nonconducted PAC

A second-degree AV block type 1 is easily confused with a nonconducted PAC (Figure 9.3).

Here is how to differentiate these conditions:

- **P Waves:** Both have P waves that are not followed by a QRS complex. However, P waves in the second-degree AV block type 1 are a sinus P wave. P wave in nonconducted PAC is a nonsinus P wave because the impulse is generated by an ectopic source rather than the SA node. Sinus P waves are upright and rounded, and look like the other P waves in the rhythm; a nonconducted P wave is different in morphology, such as notched, flattened, or peaked.

- **PR Interval:** The second-degree AV block type 1 has a progressively lengthening PR interval that is in constant sinus rhythm. The nonconducted PAC does not have a PR interval, because there is no QRS.

- **P-to-P Interval:** The second-degree AV block type 1 has regular P-to-P intervals, whereas the P wave in the nonconducted PAC condition comes earlier in the cardiac cycle.

Cause of a Second-Degree AV Block Type 1

A second-degree AV block type 1 can occur in healthy individuals, most often during sleep without the patient realizing the blockage has occurred. This blockage can also occur in a myocardial infarction involving the inferior cardiac wall, which usually resolves itself within three days. Other causes of a second-degree AV block type 1 are:

- **Medication:** Medications that slow the conduction through the AV node, beta blockers, and calcium channel blockers.

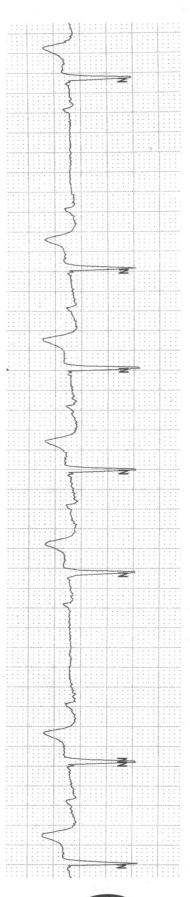

2° heart block
not followed
by

Figure 9.2 Wenckebach, or second-degree type 1, block.

133

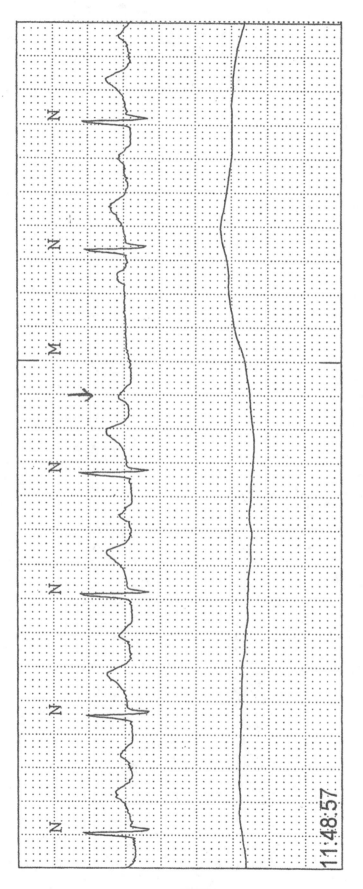

11:48:57

Figure 9.3 Nonconducted PAC.

- **Vagal Tone:** Increased impulses along the vagus nerve reduce cardiac impulses. Once stimulation to the vagus nerve stops, normal cardiac impulses return.

- **Hyperkalemia:** Abnormally high levels of potassium can decrease cardiac conductivity.

- **Cardiac Inflammation:** Myocarditis and endocarditis are secondary to inflammation of the cardiac conductive pathways.

- **Age:** The cardiac conduction system degenerates with age.

Treatment of a Second-Degree AV Block Type 1

A second-degree AV block type 1 is treated only when the patient becomes symptomatic. Treatment includes:

- In an emergency, in which the patient is hemodynamically unstable with bradycardia, the patient is administered atropine. Atropine works by speeding up the rate of the SA node, not by speeding conduction through the AV node. For symptomatic bradycardia, the dose of atropine is 0.5 to 1.0 mg by IV push, may repeat every 3 to 5 minutes up to a maximum dose of 3.0 mg.

- Medication might be changed or discontinued if the medication is the cause of the second-degree AV block type 1.

- A pacemaker is inserted if the patient experiences congestive heart failure, presyncope with pauses, or the patient feels as though she is going to pass out when she drops a QRS or if the second-degree AV block type 1 occurs after open heart surgery and other treatments fail to resolve the blockage.

9.6   Second-Degree AV Block Type 2

A second-degree type 2 AV block, referred to as *classical* or *Mobitz 2,* is less common and more serious than a type 1 second-degree AV block. The difference between a type 1 and type 2 is that the block in a type 1 is in the AV node. In a type 2, the block is infranodal between the AV node and the bundle of His and bundle branches. The patient may or may not be symptomatic. The patient may progress to third-degree AV block or ventricular standstill with little or no warning.

Definition of a Second-Degree AV Block Type 2

A second-degree AV block type 2 (Figure 9.4) is defined on the ECG as:

- **P Wave:** There are more P waves than QRS complexes such as three or four P waves to each QRS complex. If there are two P waves per QRS complex it is difficult to differentiate between a type 1 and a type 2 second-degree AV blockage. (Hint: Measure the PR interval. If it is progressively lengthening, it is a second-degree type 1 block.)

- **PR Interval:** The PR interval may be 0.12 to 0.20 seconds (normal) or prolonged. However, the PR interval remains constant, which distinguishes it from the second-degree AV block type 1, in which the PR interval progressively lengthens.

- **P-to-P Interval:** The second-degree AV block type 2 has regular P-to-P intervals.

- **QRS Complex:** The QRS complex is wide if the blockage is located in the bundle branches and is narrow if the blockage is in the bundle of His.

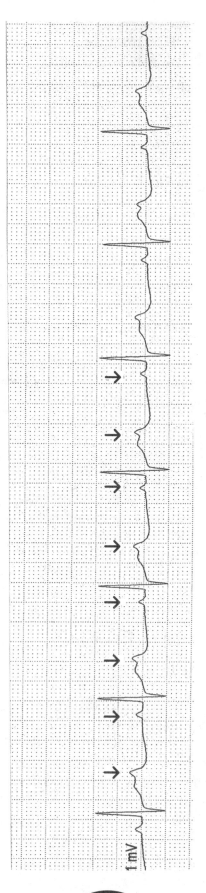

Figure 9.4 Second-degree AV block type 2, with 2:1 conduction.

Cause of a Second-Degree AV Block Type 2

A second-degree AV block type 2 is not caused by increased vagal tone or medication. It can be caused by:

- **Myocardial Infarction:** Involving the inferior cardiac wall
- **Age:** The cardiac conduction system degenerates with age
- **Cardiac Inflammation:** Myocarditis secondary to inflammation of the cardiac conductive pathways

Treatment of a Second-Degree AV Block Type 2

Treatment of a second-degree AV block type 2 includes:

- In an emergency in which the patient is hemodynamically unstable with bradycardia, the patient is administered atropine. Atropine works by speeding up the rate of the SA node through vagolytic effects. However, using it with a block in the His-Purkinje system may precipitate a third-degree block.
- A pacemaker is inserted if there is a wide QRS complex, indicating a conductivity problem with the bundle branches regardless of whether the patient is asymptomatic.

9.7   Third-Degree AV Block

A third-degree AV block occurs when there is no conduction between the AV node and the ventricles—there is a complete heart block. This is an emergency situation. The patient may report the following symptoms because of a slow ventricular rate and loss of the atrial kick:

- Syncope (Stokes-Adams syncope)—fainting caused by cardiac arrhythmia
- Fatigue
- Dizziness
- Hypotension
- Chest pain
- Dyspnea—difficulty breathing

A third-degree AV block occurs when:

- **Atria:** These are depolarized by the SA node at a rate between 60 and 100 bpm.
- **Ventricles:** These are depolarized by an escape pacemaker site. If the rate is between 40 and 60 bpm, then the location of the escape pacemaker site is in the junctional area. If the rate is between 30 and 40 bpm, then the location of the escape pacemaker site is in the ventricles.

A third-degree AV block (Figure 9.5) is defined as:

- **PR Interval:** None.
- **P-to-P Interval:** The third-degree AV block has regular P-to-P intervals.
- **QRS Complex:** The QRS complex is wide and a rate <40 bpm if the blockage is located in the bundle branches (chronic complete heart block) and is narrow and the rate is between 40 and 60 bpm if the blockage is in the bundle of His (acute complete heart block).

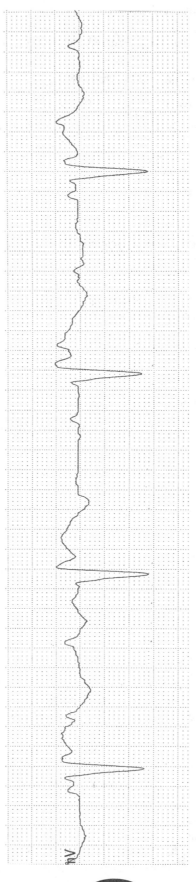

Figure 9.5 Complete heart block with a ventricular response of 30.

Causes of a Third-Degree AV Block

The causes of a third-degree AV block depend on whether the complete heart block is acute or chronic. Acute causes of third-degree heart block (narrow QRS complex) include:

- **Myocardial Infarction:** Involving the inferior cardiac wall

- **Ischemic Heart Disease**

- **Cardiac Inflammation:** Myocarditis secondary to inflammation of the cardiac conductive pathways

- **Medication:** Beta blockers, calcium channel blockers, or medications that either slow or block conduction of the AV node

- **Hyperkalemia:** Abnormal high levels of potassium can decrease cardiac conductivity

Chronic Causes of a Third-Degree Heart Block (Wide QRS Complex)

- Age: The cardiac conduction system degenerates with age.

- Acute myocardial infarction.

Treatment of a Third-Degree AV Block

A third-degree AV block requires emergency treatment. The patient requires transcutaneous pacing in which an external pacemaker is attached to the patient's chest wall. This is performed while the patient is being prepared for a transvenous pacemaker.

If the patient has a narrow QRS complex, then he or she is administered atropine. Atropine works by speeding up the rate of the SA node, not by speeding conduction through the AV node.

If the patient has a wide QRS complex, then atropine is not administered. (See Chapter 12 for further emergency treatment.)

Solved Problems

Atrioventricular Blocks

9.1   What is the normal conduction of cardiac impulse?

Normal conduction of the cardiac impulse is initiated by the SA node and travels through the atria to the AV node. From the AV node, the cardiac impulse travels through the bundle of His, then to the bundle branches, and finally to the ventricles.

9.2   How does conduction of the cardiac impulse in an AV heart block differ from normal conduction?

In an AV heart block, the impulse is either delayed or terminated before the ventricles are depolarized.

9.3   What is the normal PR interval?

In a normal cardiac impulse, the PR interval is between 0.12 and 0.20 seconds.

9.4   What are changes for the PR interval in an AV block?

- A PR interval >0.20 seconds.

- Variation in the PR interval in which the interval progressively becomes longer.

- No PR interval. There is no relationship between the P wave and the QRS complex.

9.5   What are the categories of an AV blockage?

The three degrees of AV blockage are:

- **First-Degree:** Less harmful

- **Second-Degree:** Divided into two types

    o   Type 1

    o   Type 2

- **Third-Degree:** Complete heart block (CHB)

9.6   What is Mobitz 2?

Mobitz 2 is a type 2 second-degree AV block.

9.7   How does a first-degree AV block appear on an ECG?

- **P Wave:** There is one P wave for every QRS complex.

- **PR Interval:** The P wave is delayed in the AV node longer than normal, resulting in a prolonged PR interval >0.20.

- **QRS Complex:** The QRS complex is normal because every P wave is conducted through to the ventricles.

9.8   How does a myocardial ischemia or infarct in the inferior wall of the heart cause a first-degree AV block?

A first-degree AV block can also occur in a myocardial ischemia or infarct in the inferior wall of the heart. The right coronary artery supplies 90% of the blood to the AV node. Likewise, the circumflex artery supplies the AV node with 10% of its blood supply. If either or both of these arteries narrows, blood supply to the AV node decreases, therefore reducing the AV node cardiac impulse.

9.9   How can the vagal tone cause a first-degree AV block?

A first-degree AV block might occur in a healthy person when there is an increased vagal tone. That is, increased impulses along the vagus nerve reduce cardiac impulses. Once stimulation to the vagus nerve stops, normal cardiac impulses return.

9.10   How does endocarditis cause a first-degree AV block?

The cardiac conduction pathways become infected.

9.11   How can age cause a first-degree AV block?

The cardiac conduction system degenerates with age.

9.12   How can hyperkalemia cause a first-degree AV block?

Hyperkalemia, which is an abnormally high level of potassium in the blood, can decrease cardiac conductivity.

9.13   What is the treatment for first-degree AV block?

A first-degree AV block is usually asymptomatic. The patient likely does not realize there is decreased AV node conductivity. Therefore, there is no treatment required for first-degree AV block.

9.14   Why might a health care provider monitor a patient who has a first-degree AV block?

If a health care provider identifies a first-degree AV block during a routine examination, the health care provider is likely to monitor the patient's cardiac conductivity regularly since a first-degree AV block may progress to more symptomatic AV blocks.

9.15   What is a Wenckebach block?

A second-degree type 1 AV block is referred to as a Wenckebach block.

9.16   What is nearly always the cause of a second-degree type 1 AV block?

The second-degree type 1 AV block is nearly always caused by a disease of the AV node.

9.17   What would you explain to a patient who has been diagnosed with a second-degree type 1 AV block?

This type of AV block is seldom serious; however, it can progress to a more serious AV block. The patient may report feeling an irregular heartbeat.

9.18   How would a second-degree type 1 AV block appear on an ECG?

The atrial rhythm is regular and the ventricular rhythm is irregular. It is defined on the ECG as:

- **P Wave:** Some P waves are not followed by a QRS complex.

- **P-to-P Interval:** The distance between P waves is regular.

- **PR Interval:** The PR interval progressively lengthens because the impulse is held increasingly longer at the AV node until one impulse is not conducted through to the ventricles. This results in a nonconducted P wave, occasioning a pause that causes an atrial, junctional, or ventricular escape beat during the pause. Once the cardiac cycle is completed (lengthening of the PR interval and dropped beat), the cardiac cycle starts over. This is represented by a group of beats on the ECG.

- **QRS Complex:** The QRS complex represents cardiac impulses that are conducted through the AV node and are <0.10 seconds on the ECG.

9.19   How do you differentiate between second-degree type 1 AV block and a nonconducted PAC?

- **P Waves:** Both have P waves that are not followed by a QRS complex. However, P waves in the second-degree type 1 AV block are a sinus P wave. P wave in nonconducted PAC is a nonsinus P wave because the impulse is generated by an ectopic source rather than the SA node.

- **PR Interval:** The second-degree type 1 AV block has a progressively lengthening PR interval that is in constant sinus rhythm.

- **P-to-P Interval:** The second-degree type 1 AV block has regular P-to-P intervals, whereas the P wave in the nonconducted PAC condition comes earlier in the cardiac cycle.

9.20   Where is the blockage if the patient with a second-degree type 2 AV block shows a narrow QRS complex?

The blockage is in the bundle of His.

9.21   What is a feature in the ECG that distinguishes a second-degree type 1 AV block from a second-degree type 2 AV block?

The PR interval may be between 0.12 to 0.20 seconds (normal) or prolonged. However, the PR interval remains constant, which distinguishes it from a second-degree type 1 AV block, in which the PR interval progressively lengthens.

9.22   What are treatments for second-degree type 2 AV block?

In an emergency in which the patient is hemodynamically unstable with bradycardia, the patient is administered atropine. A pacemaker is inserted if there is a wide QRS complex indicating a conductivity problem with the bundle branches, regardless of whether the patient is asymptomatic.

9.23   How does atropine affect a second-degree type 2 AV block?

Atropine works by speeding up the rate of the SA node, not by speeding conduction through the AV node.

9.24   What is Stokes-Adams syncope?

Stokes-Adams syncope is fainting caused by cardiac arrhythmia.

9.25   What is a third-degree AV block?

A third-degree AV block occurs when there is no conduction between the AV node and the ventricles—there is a complete heart block. This is an emergency situation.

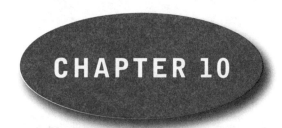

CHAPTER 10

Ventricular Arrhythmias and Bundle Branch Blocks

10.1 Definition

Blockage of either the left or right bundle branches results in depolarization of the ventricles through a different conduction pathway. Normal conduction through the bundle branches occurs simultaneously, resulting in concurrent depolarization of both the right and left ventricles. With a bundle branch block, one ventricle depolarizes before the other, resulting in a notched QRS. The rate is usually that of the underlying rhythm. Differentiating between a right and left requires a 12-lead ECG.

Ventricular arrhythmias are caused by a number of conditions. These are:

- **Altered or Enhanced Automaticity:** This occurs when cardiac cells in the ventricles have a lower than normal threshold for stimulus, which is seen in hyperkalemia.

- **Triggered Activity:** This results from abnormal depolarizations of cardiac cells, called after-depolarizations. Triggered activity is seen in patients with digitoxin toxicity and in the reperfusion arrhythmia that follows a myocardial infarction.

- **Re-entry:** This is an accessory conduction pathway that allows the impulse to travel in a circle instead of a top-to-bottom pathway.

10.2 Premature Ventricular Contractions (PVC)

Premature ventricular contractions are extra beats that originate either in the right or left ventricles early in the cardiac cycle. This is caused by an ectopic impulse site located below the bundle of His.

Premature beats are graded using the Lown grading system. The higher the grade, the more serious is the condition. The grading scale follows:

- Grade 0 = No premature beats

- Grade 1 = Occasional (<30/h)

- Grade 2 = Frequent (>30/h)

- Grade 3 = Multiform
- Grade 4 = Repetitive (A = Couplets, B = Salvos of ≥ 3)
- Grade 5 = R-on-T pattern

Premature Ventricular Contractions: ECG

Premature ventricular contractions (Figure 10.1) have the following characteristics on an ECG:

- **QRS Complex:** Width >0.12 seconds. Takes on a bizarre and abnormal appearance compared with the underlying rhythm.
- **Underlying Rhythm:** Regular except for interruptions of PVC and subsequent pause, which makes the rhythm irregular.
- **P Wave:** No P wave is associated with the PVC.
- **PR Interval:** No PR interval is present.
- **T Wave:** Opposite deflection from the main deflection. Repolarization is abnormal.

Premature Ventricular Contractions: Pauses

A pause follows a premature ventricular contraction. The pause can be:

- **Compensatory (typical):** A compensatory pause occurs because the SA node is not depolarized by the PVC. This is characterized as:
  - The time between the R waves that occur before and after the PVC is equal to the R-R interval of the underlying regular rhythm.
- **Noncompensatory:** A noncompensatory pause occurs because the PVC depolarizes the SA node. This is characterized as:
  - The time between the R waves that occur before and after the PVC is not equal to the R-R interval of the underlying regular rhythm.

Premature Ventricular Contraction Naming Conventions

A PVC (Figure 10.2) is identified by its frequency. Here are some terms used to identify a PVC:

- **Rare PVC:** There are fewer than six PVCs per minute.
- **Frequent PVC:** There are six or more PVCs per minute.
- **Bigeminy:** PVC occurs with every other contraction.
- **Trigeminy:** PVC occurs with every third contraction.
- **Quadrigeminy:** PVC occurs with every fourth contraction.
- **Couplet (Paired):** PVCs occur back to back.

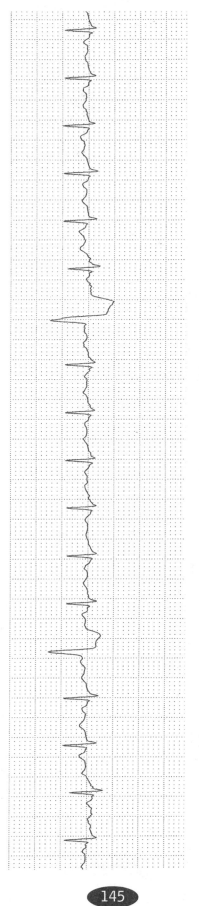

Figure 10.1 NSR with two unifocal PVCs, fifth beat and twelfth beat.

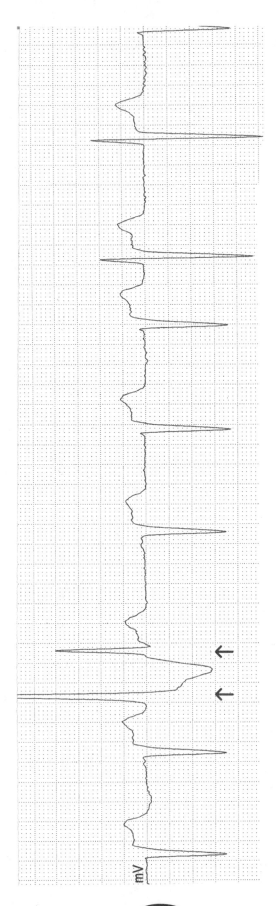

Figure 10.2 Premature ventricular contractions.

- **Triplet:** PVC occurs in a set of three.
- **Ventricular Tachycardia (Burst of V-Tach, Run of V-Tach, Paroxysmal):** This is PVC occurring in a set greater than three (Figure 10.3).

Premature Ventricular Contractions: Foci

A premature ventricular contraction is also described in relation to the foci (number) of the ectopic impulse site that is causing the PVC. These are called:

- **Unifocal:** There is one ectopic impulse site that is causing the PVC. Each PVC looks the same on the ECG.
- **Multifocal:** There are multiple ectopic impulse sites causing the PVC. PVCs look different on the ECG because each might be caused by a different ectopic site.

Premature Ventricular Contractions: The R-on-T Phenomenon

The R-on-T phenomenon occurs when the premature ventricular contraction (Grade V PVC) occurs during the relative refractory period. It is at this time that the ventricles are recovering from contraction and are represented on the ECG as the T wave.

When the ventricular ectopic site sends an impulse (represented as the R wave on the ECG), the ventricles are stimulated to contract, although the ventricles still have not recovered from the previous contraction stimulated by the underlying rhythm. This is depicted on the ECG as a ventricular rhythm beginning from the middle of the T wave.

This is the most vulnerable time for the ventricles and can lead to tachycardia (rhythm >180 bpm) or ventricular fibrillation, which is the fluttering of the ventricles leading to cardiac arrest.

Causes of Premature Ventricular Contractions

There are four common causes of PVC:

1. **Cardiac Disease:**
   a. Acute myocardial infarction
   b. Cardiac ischemia
   c. Myocarditis (inflammation of the cardiac tissue and cells)
   d. Cardiomyopathies
   e. Myocardial contusion
   f. Valve disease, especially mitral valve

2. **Medications:**
   a. Tricyclic antidepressants (such as amitriptyline or nortriptyline) interacting with quinidines
   b. Digoxin at toxic levels
   c. Sympathomimetics, epinephrine
   d. Aminophylline
   e. Caffeine

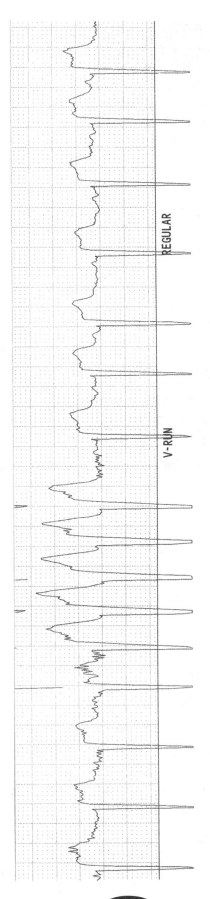

Figure 10.3 Four-beat run of v-tach, or ventricular tachycardia.

3. **Hormones:**

   a. Increase catecholamines through emotional stress or use of drugs (cocaine, amphetamines, alcohol, tobacco)

4. **Medical Conditions:**

   a. Hypokalemia

   b. Hypomagnesemia

   c. Hypoxia

   d. Hypercapnia

Treatment of Premature Ventricular Contractions

Treatment of PVC depends on a number of factors:

- **Grade 1 PVC:** No treatment is necessary if the patient is relatively healthy.

- **Grade 2 PVC:** Occasional <30/min unifocal, if asymptomatic no treatment is necessary, consider treating the underlying causes such as electrolyte imbalances, avoiding triggers such as caffeine. Use Digibind for digitoxin toxicity, and a 12-lead ECG to rule out ischemic disease (angioplasty may be needed).

- **Grade 3 PVC:** Frequent, 30/min, see treatment for Grade 2 PVC.

- **Grade 4/5 PVC:** Repetitive such as a bigeminy pattern, and a Grade 5 is an R-on-T. The patient is administered antiarrhythmic medications such as amiodarone and lidocaine because there is a higher mortality rate for this condition.

- Reverse the underlying cause:

  o *Hypoxia:* Administer oxygen.

  o *Heart Failure:* Encourage diuresis.

  o *Hypokalemia:* Administer potassium.

  o *Hypomagnesemia:* Administer magnesium.

  o *Myocarditis:* Administer anti-inflammatory medication.

  o *Drug Induced:* Discontinue or decrease medication.

10.3　Ventricular Tachycardia (V-Tach)

Ventricular tachycardia (Figure 10.4) is an impulse rate ≥120 bpm that is generated from one or multiple ectopic sites in the ventricles. Monomorphic ventricular tachycardia is from one ectopic site and polymorphic ventricular tachycardia is from multiple ectopic sites.

As the impulse rate increases to 250 bpm, the patient loses atrial kick and becomes hemodynamically unstable. The patient shows signs of:

- Hypotension

- Nausea

- Palpitations

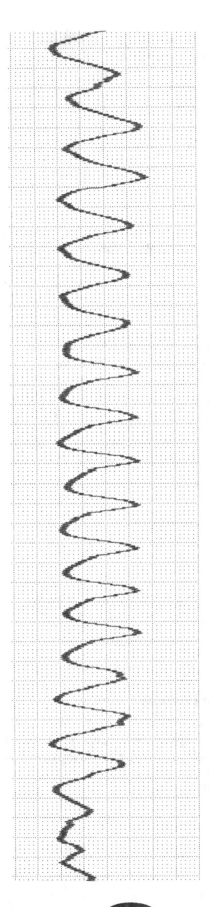

Figure 10.4 Ventricular tachycardia.

- Difficulty breathing

- Being unresponsive

Ventricular tachycardia can progress to ventricular fibrillation, in which the ventricles flutter rather than contract and repolarize. Before ventricular fibrillation, the ECG will show torsades de pointes (twisting of the pointes) in which the tracing appears to twist.

　　The health of the patient's heart determines the patient's response to ventricular tachycardia. However, ventricular tachycardia lasting <30 seconds is nonsustainable because the patient becomes hemodynamically unstable.

Ventricular Tachycardia and the ECG

Ventricular tachycardia (Figure 10.5) is identified on an ECG by the following characteristics:

- **P Wave:** The P wave is hidden within the QRS complex and might be occasionally seen between QRS complexes.

- **PR Interval:** Not measurable.

- **QRS Complex:** Wide, distorted, and bizarre.

- **Rhythm:** Regular but can be irregular.

- **Torsades de Pointes Waveform:** R-on-T phenomenon as a result of hypomagnesemia and prolonged QT intervals.

Causes of Ventricular Tachycardia

There are a number of causes of ventricular tachycardia, including heart disease, such as heart failure, and structural defects, such as mitral value disorder. The most common cause of monomorphic ventricular tachycardia is a prior myocardial infarction that resulted in the formation of myocardial scar tissue. Nonsustained ventricular tachycardia is commonly related to cardiac ischemia and acute myocardial infarction. An imbalance of a patient's electrolytes can result in ventricular tachycardia. These are hypokalemia, hypomagnesemia, and hypocalcemia.

　　Medications can trigger ventricular tachycardia. These are:

- Type 1A antiarrhythmic drugs by prolonging QT intervals

  - Quinidines

  - Procainamide

- Tikosyn

- Psychotropic Medications: TCA and phenothiazine predisposes the patient to polymorphic ventricular tachycardia (torsades de pointes)

- Cocaine

- Methamphetamines

Ventricular tachycardia can also result from irritation by a catheter inserted into the pulmonary artery in the right ventricle.

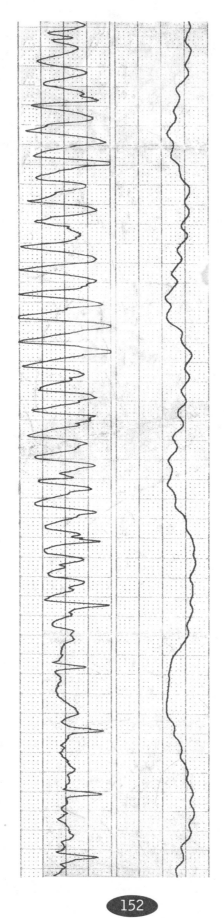

Figure 10.5 Polymorphic ventricular tachycardia, or torsades de pointes.

Treatment of Ventricular Tachycardia

Treatment of ventricular tachycardia is dependent on the characteristics of the condition. Treatments are:

- Stable monomorphic ventricular tachycardia:
  - Administer antiarrhythmics such as amiodarone, Lidocaine, and procainamide.
  - Perform cardioversion or defibrillation.
  - Rebalance electrolytes (potassium, magnesium, calcium).
- Unstable monomorphic ventricular tachycardia caused by hemodynamic instability:
  - Perform cardioversion or defibrillation.
- Chronic or recurrent ventricular tachycardia:
  - Administer antiarrhythmic.
  - Use radiofrequency ablation (destroying the ectopic site).
  - Implant an automatic implantable cardiac defibrillator (AICD).
  - Electrophysiology studies (EP) done in the EP lab with the electrophysiologist. Patient susceptibility to these lethal rhythms is tested in a controlled environment.
- Polymorphic ventricular tachycardia (torsades de pointes):
  - Rebalance electrolytes (potassium, magnesium, calcium).
  - Perform defibrillation.

10.4 Ventricular Fibrillation

Ventricular fibrillation is the quivering of the ventricles, resulting in a rhythm that cannot support perfusion of blood vessels and is the primary cause of sudden cardiac death. The patient is hemodynamically unstable. There is no cardiac output. The patient is without a pulse, without blood pressure, unresponsive, and death is imminent because ventricular fibrillation progresses to ventricular standstill or asystole.

Ventricular fibrillation has the following ECG characteristics:

- **P Wave:** None
- **QRS Complex:** None
- **PR Interval:** Not measurable
- **Wave:**
  - Fine wave (Figure 10.6) requires antiarrhythmic medication before defibrillation, as it is of longer duration.
  - Coarse wave (Figure 10.7) is likely to respond to defibrillation because it is a new onset.

Causes of Ventricular Fibrillation

Ventricular fibrillation can be caused by a number of conditions. The most common are:

- Structural heart disease:
  - Myocardial ischemia or infarction resulting from coronary artery disease.

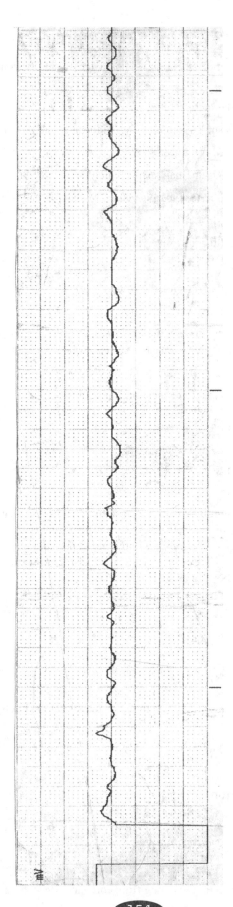

Figure 10.6 Fine ventricular fibrillation.

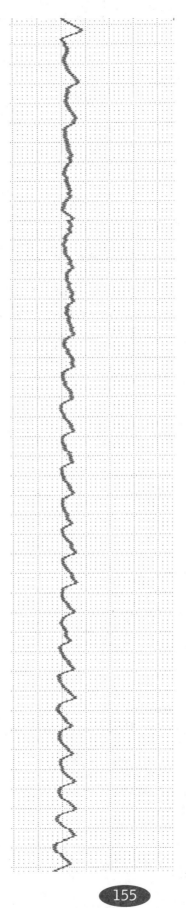

Figure 10.7 Coarse ventricular fibrillation.

- Dilated and hypertrophic cardiomyopathies are the second most important cardiac cause of sudden death.

- Aortic stenosis.

- Aortic dissection.

- Pericardial tamponade.

- Congenital heart disease.

- Myocarditis.

- Nonstructural heart condition:

    - Heart block.

    - Pre-excitation, in which ventricles become depolarized too soon.

    - Long QT syndrome, in which there is a delayed repolarization of the heart.

    - Short QT syndrome, a QT interval <300 ms, does not change with heart rate, and the heart has no structural defects. This is an inherited syndrome.

    - Electrocution.

    - Medication-induced QT prolongation with torsades de pointes, such as a drug-to-drug interaction between quinidines and tricyclic antidepressants.

    - Brugada syndrome, which is an inherited syndrome responsible for sudden cardiac death and is only detected with 12-lead ECG. Diagnosis is difficult, usually after the patient dies unexpectedly from cardiac arrest.

    - Adverse effect of inserting a catheter into the pulmonary artery, such as placement of a pacemaker.

- Hypoxia

    - Aspiration

    - Sleep apnea

    - Primary pulmonary hypertension

    - Pulmonary embolism

    - Tension pneumothorax

- Metabolic Imbalance

    - Electrolyte disturbances and acidosis

- Toxins

    - Cocaine toxicity

    - Digoxin toxicity

    - Proarrhythmic toxicity

    - Sepsis

- Neurologic Conditions

  ○ Seizure

  ○ Cerebrovascular accident, such as a hemorrhage or ischemic stroke

  ○ Drowning followed by rewarming of the body

Treatment of Ventricular Fibrillation

The treatment for ventricular fibrillation depends on whether the ventricular fibrillation is witnessed.

- If witnessed:

  ○ Defibrillation is administered to the patient, followed by cardiopulmonary resuscitation (CPR). Defibrillation can be administered using:

    ▪ Automated External Defibrillator (AED): Start CPR, attach the AED, and follow instructions announced by the AED.

    ▪ Monophasic Defibrillator: Set the defibrillator to 360j and administer one shock. Continue CPR for two minutes then repeat defibrillation.

    ▪ Biphasic Defibrillator: Set the defibrillator to 200 j and administer one shock. Continue CPR for two minutes then repeat defibrillation.

  ○ IV access and intubate to open an airway after the initial shock. Continue CPR during IV access and intubation. Do not interrupt compressions to check the patient's pulse if the clinical picture does not improve.

- If not witnessed or the patient is in ventricular fibrillation for a few minutes:

  ○ Provide two minutes of CPR, and then defibrillate because defibrillation is more effective after the heart receives circulated blood as a result of CPR.

  ○ Administer antiarrhythmic medication:

    ▪ Amiodarone: 300 mg IV/IO, repeat once at 150 mg IV; if rhythm converts consider 1 mg/min IV drip over 6 hours, then 0.5 mg/min over 18 hours, max dose of 2.2 gm in 24 hours. Amiodarone slows the conduction through accessory pathways and slows heart rate to allow for full repolarization.

    ▪ Lidocaine: 1 to 1.5 mg/kg IV/IO, repeat every 5 to 10 minutes at 0.5 to 0.75 mg/kg, max dose of 3 mg/kg. If rhythm converts, consider 1 to 4 mg/min IV maintenance drip Class IB antiarrhythmic, which increases the electrical stimulation threshold of the ventricle, resulting in suppression of the automaticity of conduction.

  ○ Administer vasopressors and anticholinergic medication:

    ▪ Epinephrine: (1:10,000) 1 mg IV/IO, repeat every 3 to 5 minutes. It increases peripheral resistance via α-receptor–dependent vasoconstriction and cardiac output via its binding to β-receptors.

    ▪ Vasopressin: 40 units IV/IO once, can be used as an alternative to the first or second dose of epinephrine. As an alternate to epinephrine, vasopressin causes peripheral vasoconstriction that ultimately helps increase blood pressure.

- Continue with two minutes of CPR followed by defibrillation and medication while reversing the underlying cause of ventricular fibrillation.

- The decision to stop resuscitative efforts is made by the patient's family, the patient's living will, and/or the patient's physician.

10.5   Ventricular Standstill (Asystole)

Ventricular standstill is also known as asystole (Figure 10.9), which is a condition that occurs when there is not any ventricular depolarization, resulting in absent perfusion of the vital organs. The patient is unresponsive, not breathing, with no pulse or blood pressure. There is a poor prognosis; the survival rate is <2% (see Figure 10.9).
   This condition is characterized by the following ECG:

- **P Wave:** Absent (flat line), but may be present if the patient was in an AV block such as Mobitz 2 or third-degree block.

- **QRS Complex:** None.

- **PR Interval:** Not measurable.

Causes and Treatment of Ventricular Standstill (Asystole)

Ventricular standstill is commonly caused by the following conditions:

- Hyperkalemia

- Hypothermia

- Acidosis

- Stroke

- Pulmonary embolus (saddle embolus)

- Drug overdose (narcotics), which suppresses respiration and leads to hypoxemia

- Myocardial infarction complicated by ventricular fibrillation or ventricular tachycardia that deteriorates to asystole

- Proximal occlusion of the right coronary artery causing the SA and AV node to infarct

- An infarct that creates a block affecting both bundle branches

- Indirect lightning strike

The treatment for ventricular standstill is CPR and administering rescue medications and transcutaneous pacing. Rescue medications are:

- Epinephrine: (1:10,000) 1 mg IV/IO, repeat every 3 to 5 minutes.

- Vasopressin: 40 units IV/IO once, can be used as an alternative to the first or second dose of epinephrine.

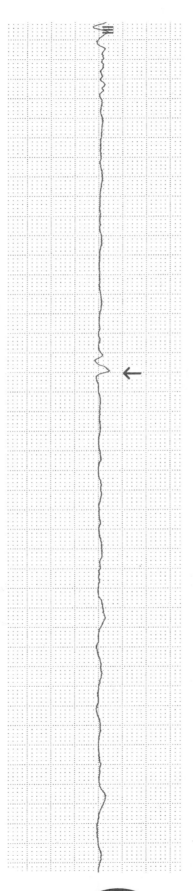

Figure 10.8 Asystole with agonal beat.

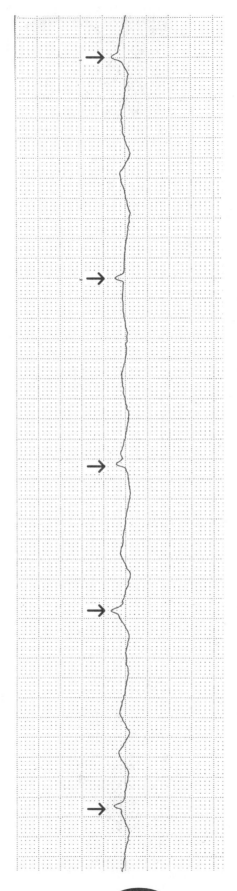

Figure 10.9 Ventricular standstill; just P waves are visible.

- Atropine: 0.03 mg/kg (dosing not to be <0.1 mg because of paradoxic bradycardia) IV/IO every three to five minutes to a total dose of 3 mg. Blocks vagal causes, resulting in increased conduction through the AV node.

10.6   Idioventricular Rhythm

An idioventricular rhythm (Figure 10.10) is a rhythm that begins in the ventricles when the ventricles are not stimulated by the SA node. The rate is between 30 and 40 bpm. An accelerated idioventricular rhythm (AIVR) (Figure 10.11) can occur, resulting in a rate between 41 and 100 bpm, which is slower than ventricular tachycardia. The patient may be asymptomatic and may tolerate an idioventricular rhythm.

Causes and Treatment of Idioventricular Rhythm

An idioventricular rhythm can be caused by:

- Myocardial ischemia or infarct, especially after an inferior myocardial infarction that affects the SA node

- Digoxin toxicity

- Hypokalemia

- Reperfusion rhythm that occurs after blood returns to an area of the heart that lacks blood flow because of an ischemia or infarction

No treatment is necessary for an idioventricular rhythm as long as the rate is adequate to perfuse the circulatory system because suppressing the ventricular rhythm might lead to a worse rhythm that reduces perfusion.

10.7   Bundle Branch Blocks

A bundle branch block occurs when transmission of the impulse from the SA node is blocked and unable to conduct through the right or left bundle branch. This results in sequential depolarization of the ventricles (depolarization at different times).

Bundle Branch Block ECG

A bundle branch block (Figure 10.12) can be detected in a single-lead ECG. However, a 12-lead ECG is required to determine if the block is from the left or right bundle branch. A bundle branch block has the following characteristics on an ECG:

- **QRS Complex:** >0.10 (wider than normal)

- **P Wave:** Normal

- **PR Interval:** 0.12 to 0.20 seconds

- **Rate:** Regular

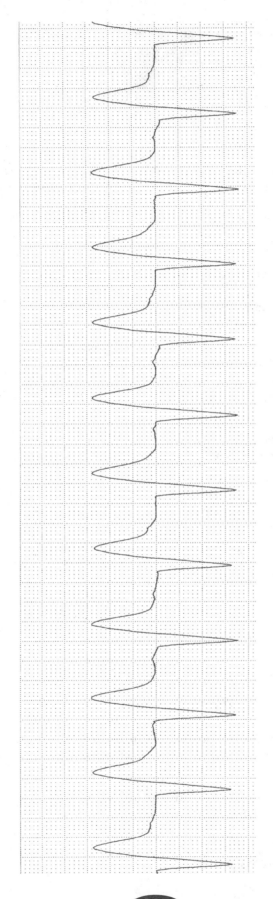

Figure 10.10 Accelerated idioventricular rhythm.

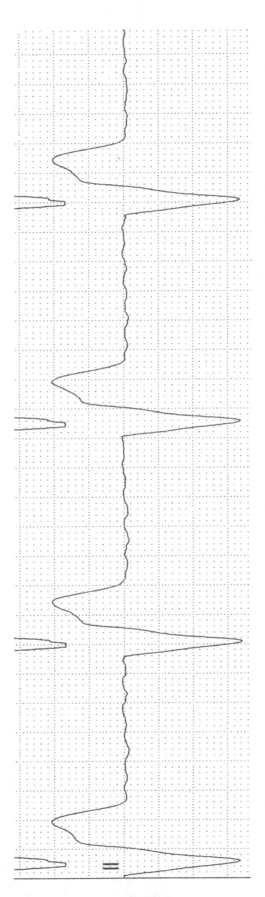

Figure 10.11 Idioventricular rhythm, rate of 42.

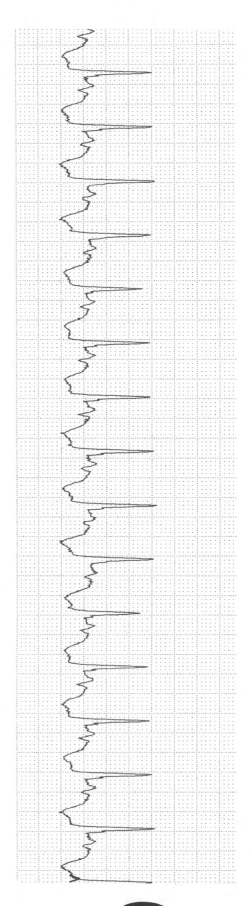

Figure 10.12 Sinus tachycardia with a bundle branch block.

Causes of Bundle Branch Block

The cause of a bundle branch block is related to whether the block is in the right bundle branch or the left bundle branch as follows:

- Right bundle branch block (RBBB)
  - Organic heart disease
    - Congenital heart disease
    - Rheumatic heart disease
  - Occurs in healthy individuals
  - Coronary heart disease
  - Hypertensive heart disease
  - Cardiomyopathy
  - Acute pulmonary embolism
- Left bundle branch block (LBBB)
  - Left ventricular hypertrophy that affects conduction through the bundle of His
  - Aortic valve replacement
  - Congenital heart defects
  - Myocardial ischemia

Treatment of Bundle Branch Block

The patient who is diagnosed with bundle branch block must undergo a full cardiac workup to assess the underlying cause.

- For patients who have presyncope or syncope, a pacemaker is the likely course of treatment.
- For patients who have congestive heart failure (CHF), the physician will consider implanting a biventricular pacemaker that synchronizes ventricular depolarization.

Solved Problems

Ventricular Arrhythmias and Bundle Branch Block

10.1   What is a bundle branch blockage?

Blockage of the bundle branches results in either right or left ventricular depolarization by an alternate conduction pathway.

10.2   What is the impact of a bundle branch block?

The impact of a bundle branch block is abnormal contractions of the ventricles called *ventricular arrhythmia*.

10.3 What causes ventricular arrhythmias?

Altered or enhanced automaticity, triggered activity, and re-entry cause ventricular arrhythmias.

10.4 What is enhanced automaticity?

Altered or enhanced automaticity occurs when cardiac cells in the ventricles have a lower than normal threshold for stimulus, which is seen in hyperkalemia.

10.5 What is a triggered activity?

Triggered activity results from abnormal depolarization of cardiac cells called *after-depolarization*. Triggered activity is seen is in patients with digitoxin toxicity and in the reperfusion arrhythmia that follows a myocardial infarction.

10.6 What are premature ventricular contractions?

Premature ventricular contractions are extra beats that originate in either the right or left ventricles early in the cardiac cycle.

10.7 What causes premature ventricular contractions?

Premature ventricular contractions are caused by an ectopic impulse site located below the bundle of His.

10.8 What is the Lown grading system?

Premature beats are graded using the Lown grading system. The higher the grade, the more serious is the condition. The grading scale is:

- Grade 0 = No premature beats
- Grade 1 = Occasional (<30/h)
- Grade 2 = Frequent (>30/h)
- Grade 3 = Multiform
- Grade 4 = Repetitive (A = couplets, B = salvos of ≥ 3)
- Grade 5 = R-on-T pattern

10.9 What naming convention is used to describe premature ventricular contractions?

- **Rare PVC:** There are less than six PVCs per minute.
- **Frequent PVC:** There are six or more PVCs per minute.
- **Bigeminy:** PVC occurs with every other contraction.
- **Trigeminy:** PVC occurs with every third contraction.
- **Quadrigeminy:** PVC occurs with every fourth contraction.
- **Couplet (Paired):** PVC occurs back to back.
- **Triplet:** PVC occurs in a set of three.
- **Ventricular Tachycardia** (burst of V-Tach, run of V-Tach, paroxysmal): PVC occurrs in a set greater than three.

10.10   What is multifocal?

Multifocal means that there are multiple ectopic impulse sites causing the PVC. PVCs look different on the ECG because each might be caused by a different ectopic site.

10.11   What is the R-on-T phenomenon?

The R-on-T phenomenon occurs when the premature ventricular contraction happens during repolarization of the ventricles of the underlying rhythm. It is at this time that the ventricles are recovering from contraction and are represented on the ECG as the T wave.

10.12   What is the treatment for Grade 1 PVC?

No treatment is necessary if the patient is relatively healthy.

10.13   What is the treatment for Grade 4/5 PVC?

To treat Grade 4/5 PVC, the patient is administered antiarrhythmic medications such as amiodarone and lidocaine because there is a higher mortality rate for this condition.

10.14   What is ventricular tachycardia?

Ventricular tachycardia is an impulse rate of 120 bpm or greater that is generated from one or multiple ectopic sites in the ventricles.

10.15   What happens when the impulse rate of ventricular tachycardia reaches 250 bpm?

As the impulse rate increases to 250 bpm, the patient loses atrial kick and becomes hemodynamically unstable.

10.16   How do you know if the patient is progressing from ventricular tachycardia to ventricular fibrillation?

Ventricular fibrillation is a chaotic rythm with no discernible complexes, whereas ventricular tachycardia has complexes that can be counted.

10.17   What would you see on an ECG if the patient is in ventricular tachycardia?

Ventricular tachycardia is identified on an ECG by the following characteristics:

- **P Wave:** The P wave is hidden within the QRS complex and might be seen occasionally between QRS complexes.

- **PR Interval:** Not measurable

- **QRS Complex:** Wide, distorted, and bizarre

- **Rhythm:** Regular but can be irregular

10.18   How would you treat stable monomorphic ventricular tachycardia?

Treat stable monomorphic ventricular tachycardia by:

- Administering antiarrhythmics such as amiodarone, lidocaine, and procainamide

- Cardioversion or defibrillation

- Rebalancing electrolytes (potassium, magnesium, calcium)

10.19   What is ventricular fibrillation?

Ventricular fibrillation is the quivering of the ventricles, resulting in a rhythm that cannot support perfusion of blood vessels and is the primary cause of sudden cardiac death.

10.20   What would you expect to see on the ECG if a patient has ventricular fibrillation?

- **P Wave:** None
- **QRS Complex:** None
- **PR Interval:** Not measurable
- **Wave:**
  - A coarse wave is likely to respond to defibrillation because it is a new onset.
  - A fine wave requires antiarrhythmic medication before defibrillation because it is of longer duration.

10.21   What are the structural heart disease causes of ventricular fibrillation?

The structural heart disease causes of ventricular fibrillation are:

- Myocardial ischemia or infarction resulting from coronary artery disease
- Dilated and hypertrophic cardiomyopathies are the second most important cardiac cause of sudden death.
- Aortic stenosis
- Aortic dissection
- Pericardial tamponade
- Congenital heart disease
- Myocarditis

10.22   What is ventricular standstill?

Ventricular standstill, also known as *asystole,* is a condition that occurs when there is no ventricular depolarization, resulting in any perfusion of the circulatory system. The patient is unresponsive, not breathing, with no pulse or blood pressure. There is a poor prognosis; the survival rate is <2%.

10.23   What is the treatment for ventricular standstill?

Treatment for ventricular standstill is cardiopulmonary resuscitation (CPR) and administering rescue medications and transcutaneous pacing. Rescue medications are:

- **Epinephrine:** (1:10,000) 1 mg IV/IO, repeat every 3 to 5 minutes.
- **Vasopressin:** 40 units IV/IO once, can be used as an alternative to the first or second dose of epinephrine.
- **Atropine:** 0.03 mg/kg (dosing not to be <0.1 mg because of paradoxic bradycardia) IV/IO, repeat every 3 to 5 minutes to a total dose of 3 mg.

10.24   What is idioventricular rhythm?

An idioventricular rhythm is one that begins in the ventricles when the ventricles are not stimulated by the SA node.

10.25   How do you differentiate between a left and right bundle branch?

A 12-lead ECG is required to determine if the block is from the left or right bundle branch.

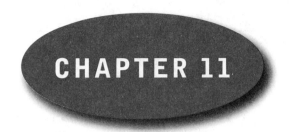

CHAPTER 11

Pacemakers

11.1 Definition

A pacemaker is an electronic, battery-operated device that monitors cardiac activity. When an abnormal rhythm or no rhythm is detected, the pacemaker sends a pulse of electricity to the heart causing cardiac muscles to contract and re-establish a perfusing rhythm. The pacemaker is connected to the heart by wires connected to one or more electrodes. An electrode is an element placed directly into the cardiac muscle.

Newer pacemakers monitor blood temperature, breathing, and cardiac electrical activity, and store this information in the pacemaker's memory, which can then be transferred to a computer for review by the health care provider.

The health care provider can program the pacemaker to modify the data monitored by the pacemaker and the response of the pacemaker to abnormal cardiac conditions. The health care provider can adjust:

- Sensitivity of the impulse in m illivolts
- When to send the impulse

There are two categories of pacemakers:

- **Internal:** The pacemaker is implanted into the patient's chest.
- **External:** The pacemaker is outside the patient's body.

There are three types of external pacemakers:

1. **Transcutaneous (TCP):** Pads containing electrodes are placed on the patient's chest. The pads are connected via wires to the pacemaker.

2. **Transvenous:** Electrode wires are placed into a vein and into either the right atrium or right ventricle. The wires are connected to the pacemaker. This is used until an internal pacemaker is implanted.

3. **Epicardial:** Electrodes are placed on the outer wall of the ventricle (epicardium) during open heart surgery. The electrodes are connected via wires to the pacemaker.

11.2 Pacemaker Function

A pacemaker can send an impulse to the heart either on a fixed rate or demand rate depending on the patient's condition and the health care provider's treatment plan for the patient.

- **Fixed Rate:** At the fixed-rate setting, the pacemaker delivers an impulse to the heart at a set rate regardless of the patient's condition. The pacemaker does not sense the patient's intrinsic cardiac activity. The pacemaker competes with the patient's own heart rate. This increases the risk of the R-on-T phenomenon. Fixed rate is commonly used in transcutaneous pacing in emergency conditions.

- **Demand Rate:** At the demand-rate setting, the pacemaker senses the patient's cardiac rhythm and delivers an impulse when the pacemaker senses no intrinsic activity. For example, a pacemaker-generated impulse is sent if the patient's natural heart rate falls below 50 bpm. Demand rate is commonly used in an internal pacemaker.

Types of Demand-Rate Pacemakers

- **Single Chamber:** The pacemaker senses and paces the atria or ventricles.

- **Dual Chamber:** The pacemaker is able to sense and pace both the atria and ventricles, thereby simulating natural AV synchronization. This preserves the atrial kick.

11.3 Transcutaneous Pacing

Transcutaneous pacing is also referred to as *external pacing* because the pacemaker's electrodes are located outside the patient's body. Transcutaneous pacing is used as a temporary solution to maintaining a sinus rhythm until transvenous pacing is implemented or transcutaneous pacing is no longer indicated

Electrodes are placed on the anterior and posterior chest walls. The pacemaker then sends an impulse over wires to the electrodes. The impulse is conducted through the chest wall to the myocardium, stimulating the heart.

Transcutaneous pacing is the initial pacing method in cardiac emergencies and is in standby mode if a patient is at risk of decompensation, such as experiencing progressively longer pauses in cardiac rhythm or having a risk of progressing to a higher degree of heart block.

When to Use Transcutaneous Pacing

Transcutaneous pacing is used when a patient:

- Is experiencing hemodynamically unstable bradycardia that does not response to atropine

- Has a type II second-degree AV block

- Has new onset bundle branch block related to an acute myocardial infarction

- Has a bundle branch block with a first-degree AV block

  - *QRS complex:* Wide

  - *T Wave:* Tall and broad

Facts About Transcutaneous Pacing

Here are a number of factors to consider when using transcutaneous pacing:

- The patient should be sedated if he or she is conscious because transcutaneous pacing is painful.
- Use large electrode pads to reduce the risk of burning the skin.
- The amount of milliamperes (mA) required to capture (contract the heart) varies depending on the patient. Lower milliamperes are required for cachectic or skinny patients. Higher milliamperes are required for obese patients or those with large muscle mass.
- Apply the minimum amount of milliamperes and increase the amount until the patient responds to pacing.
- Continue to monitor the patient to assess the clinical response to pacing. The patient's blood pressure and mentation should improve.
- Start at the pacing rate that produces improved clinical status of the patient. This decreases myocardial oxygen consumption (MVO2) and prevents further myocardial damage.

When Not to Use Transcutaneous Pacing

Transcutaneous pacing is not used in bradycardia secondary to the following conditions because conduction is not the problem:

- The heart cannot contract.
- Ischemia: Injured muscles may not be able to contract; the sodium-potassium pump is not working.
- Hypoxia: Oxygen is not available for metabolism and energy production; the patient becomes acidotic.
- Pulseless electrical activity (PEA).

11.4 Transvenous Pacing

Transvenous pacing is used as a temporary solution to the patient's cardiac conduction problem until the health care provider is able to implant a permanent pacemaker. Transvenous pacing is a less invasive procedure compared with an implanted pacemaker because the pacemaker's electrode wires are passed through a vein and inserted in the right atria, right ventricle, or both. Health care providers prefer to insert the electrode into the right ventricle because ventricular pacing is more reliable than atrial pacing due to the difficulty in placing the electrodes into the atria. Furthermore, transvenous pacing requires fewer milliamperes to contract cardiac muscle than other external pacing methods because the electrodes are directly connected to the endocardium.

Electrodes are placed through one of the following veins:

- Internal jugular vein
- Subclavian vein
- Antecubital vein
- Femoral vein

Transvenous pacing is used when the patient requires demand-rate pacing to treat symptomatic bradycardia or complete heart block with slow ventricular response. However, transvenous pacing is not useful when there are no cardiac contractions or contractions are impaired due to a drug overdose, hypoxemia, or acidosis.

11.5 Epicardial Pacing

Epicardial pacing is used during open heart surgery to maintain or re-establish cardiac rhythm. Electrodes are placed on the atria and the ventricles enabling dual-chamber sensing and pacing. Wires connecting to electrodes exit through the chest wall and connect to a cable attached to the external pacemaker. As with transvenous pacing, epicardial pacing requires fewer milliamperes to contract cardiac muscle than other external pacemakers because electrodes connect directly to the endocardium. The epicardial pacemaker is able to sense intrinsic activity and provide a demand-rate impulse as required by the patient's condition.

Epicardial pacing is used for emergency pacing when the patient has symptomatic bradycardia and heart blocks. The health care provider may place the epicardial pacemaker on standby at a lower than intrinsic rate if the patient is likely to become symptomatic. The health care provider may use epicardial pacing to improve the patient's cardiac output by manipulating the patient's heart rate.

11.6 Permanent Pacing

Permanent pacing occurs when a pacemaker is implanted in the patient's chest. The health care provider weighs the benefits and risks of the implant. Not all patients who have a temporary pacemaker require a permanent pacemaker.

A permanent pacemaker is implanted by an electrophysiologist in the electrophysiology lab (EP lab) under local anesthetic, conscious sedation, or both. A pulse generator is placed beneath the skin on the nondominant side of the patient. This reduces interference with the patient's normal activities. Electrodes of the permanent pacemaker are placed through the subclavian or cephalic vein into the atrium, ventricle, or both using a fluoroscopy to guide placement.

Once in place, the health care provider can initiate single- or dual-chamber pacing or AV synchronous pacing.

Biventricular pacing reduces ventricular remodeling that can result from single ventricular pacing and can improve cardiac function in patients who have congestive heart failure. In biventricular pacing one electrode is inserted into the right ventricle against the septum and another electrode is inserted in the lateral wall of the left ventricle.

Permanent pacemakers are powered by a battery that lasts 5 to 12 years. The patient and the health care provider monitor the battery condition regularly.

11.7 Pacing Terminology

Here is a list of terminology commonly used in cardiac pacing:

- **Capture** (Figure 11.1): The impulse causes the myocardium to contract.
- **Capture Threshold:** The minimum milliamperes required to capture. A QRS complex is seen on an ECG after each pacing impulse.

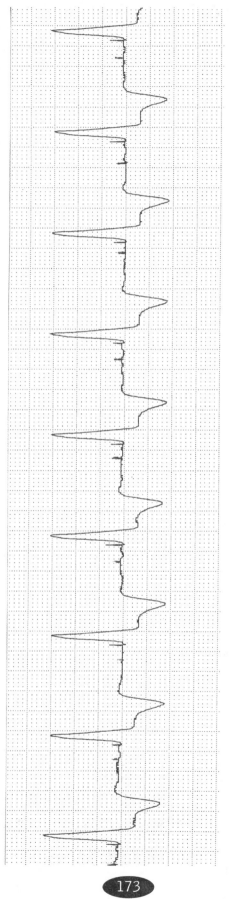

Figure 11.1 Capture one QRS for every pacemaker spike; check for 100% AV pacing and sensing appropriately.

- **Failure to Capture** (Figure 11.2): The impulse fails to contract the myocardium. There is a pacing impulse without a QRS complex. This can be caused by the following scenarios:

  ○ The impulse occurs during the absolute refractory period or the wrong point in the cardiac cycle.

  ○ High pacing thresholds caused by:

    ▪ Acidosis/alkalosis

    ▪ Hyperkalemia

    ▪ Broken wires

    ▪ Pacemaker box failure

    ▪ Bad connection to an external pulse generator

    ▪ Battery failure

    ▪ An inflammatory reaction or fibrosis at the electrode-myocardium interface

    ▪ Remedy:

      ♦ Increase the milliamperes and check all connections.

      ♦ Have the bedside monitor and transcutaneous pacing on standby in case complete failure to capture occurs.

- **Failure to Sense** (Figure 11.3): The pacemaker fails to sense intrinsic cardiac activity in demand pacing and is unable to deliver the impulse appropriately. Decreased millivolts increase sensitivity to intrinsic activity. Conversely, increased millivolts decrease sensitivity. Failure to sense can lead to an R-on-T phenomenon or failure to deliver an impulse when needed; the patient may feel symptomatic if he or she is not receiving the appropriate amount of impulses because of oversensing.

Pacemaker Modes

A pacemaker mode defines how the pacemaker is functioning. The pacemaker mode is defined by up to five letters; however, usually the first three letters describe the mode. Here is how to decode pacemaker modes:

- The first letter defines the chamber paced.

  ○ *A*—Atria

  ○ *V*—Ventricle

  ○ *D*—Dual, for both atria and ventricles

- The second letter defines the chamber being paced.

  ○ *A*—Atria

  ○ *V*—Ventricles

  ○ *D*—Dual, both atria and ventricles

  ○ *O*—None sensed

    ▪ *O* is used when pacing is not dependent on sensing electrical activity.

- The third letter is the pacemaker's programmed response to the sensing.

  ○ *I*—The pacemaker is inhibited.

  ○ *T*—The pacemaker is triggered to respond.

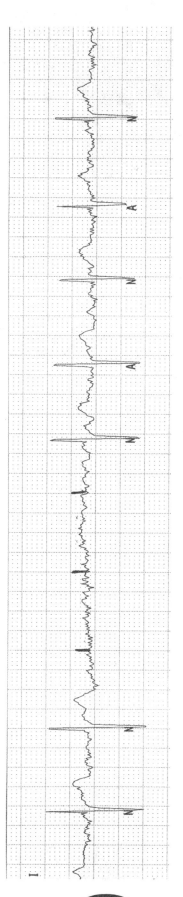

Figure 11.2 Failure to capture.

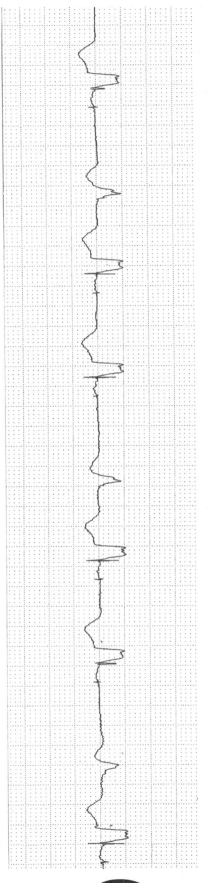

Figure 11.3 Sensing the intrinsic beats (second and fifth beats) appropriately.

- *D*—Any electrical activity by the atria or ventricles will inhibit the pacemaker; however, if the pacemaker senses any atrial activity then a *V*-paced beat will be triggered.

- *O*—None.

- The fourth letter is the programmability and rate response of the pacemaker.

   - *P*—Simple programmable

   - *M*—Multiprogrammability

   - *C*—Communication

   - *R*—Rate-response ("physiologic") pacing

   - *O*—No programmability or rate modulation

- The fifth letter relates to the antitachyarrhythmia function (Figure 11.4).

   - *P*—Pacing (antitachyarrhythmia)

   - *S*—Shock

   - *D*—Dual (pacing + shock)

Solved Problems

Pacemakers

11.1   What is a pacemaker?

A pacemaker is an electronic, battery-operated device that monitors cardiac activity. When an abnormal rhythm or no rhythm is detected, the pacemaker sends a pulse of electricity to the heart, causing cardiac muscles to contract and re-establish a perfusing rhythm.

11.2   How can a health care provider modify a pacemaker?

The health care provider can program the pacemaker to modify the data monitored by the pacemaker and the response of the pacemaker to abnormal cardiac conditions. The health care provider can adjust the sensitivity of the impulse in millivolts, and then send the impulse. Increasing the heart rate increases cardiac output.

11.3   What are the two categories of pacemakers?

- **Internal:** The pacemaker is implanted into the patient's chest.

- **External:** The pacemaker is outside the patient's body.

11.4   What are the four types of external pacemakers?

The three types of external pacemakers are transcutaneous (TCP), transvenous, and transthoracic, or epicardial.

11.5   What is a TCP pacemaker?

In a TCP pacemaker, pads containing electrodes are placed on the patient's chest. The pads are connected via wires to the pacemaker.

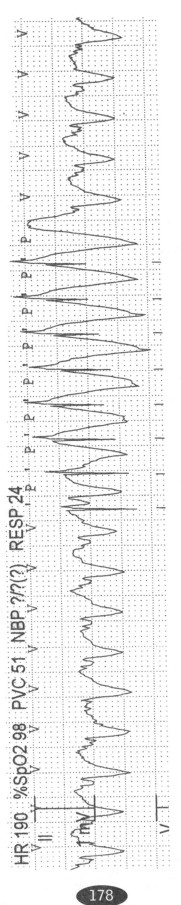

Figure 11.4 Antitachyarrhythmia function during ventricular tachycardia.

11.6   What is a transvenous pacemaker?

In a transvenous pacemaker, electrode wires are placed into a vein and into either the right atrium or right ventricle. The wires are connected to the pacemaker. This is used until an internal pacemaker is implanted.

11.7   What is an epicardial pacemaker?

In an epicardial pacemaker, electrodes are placed on the outer wall of the ventricle (epicardium) during open heart surgery. The electrodes are connected via wires to the pacemaker.

11.8   What is fixed-rate pacing?

At the fixed-rate setting, the pacemaker delivers an impulse to the heart at a set rate regardless of the patient's condition. The pacemaker does not monitor the patient's cardiac activity before, during, or after sending the impulse to the heart. The pacemaker competes with the patient's own heart rate. This increases the risk of the R-on-T phenomenon. Fixed rate is commonly used in transcutaneous pacing in emergency conditions.

11.9   What is demand-rate pacing?

At the demand-rate setting, the pacemaker senses the patient's cardiac rhythm and delivers an impulse when the pacemaker senses no intrinsic activity. For example, an impulse is sent if the patient's natural heart rate falls <50 bpm. Demand rate is commonly used in an internal pacemaker.

11.10   What is single-chamber pacing?

In single-chamber pacing, the pacemaker senses atrial activity and reacts accordingly.

11.11   What is dual-chamber pacing?

In dual-chamber pacing, the pacemaker is able to sense and pace both the atria and ventricles, thereby simulating the natural AV synchronization. This preserves the atrial kick.

11.12   Why is transcutaneous pacing performed?

Transcutaneous pacing is used as a temporary solution to maintain a sinus rhythm until either transvenous pacing is implemented or an internal permanent pacemaker is implanted into the patient.

11.13   Where are electrodes placed in transcutaneous pacing?

Electrodes are placed on the anterior and posterior chest walls.

11.14   When is transcutaneous pacing used?

Transcutaneous pacing is used when a patient:

- Is experiencing hemodynamically unstable bradycardia and does not response to atropine.
- Has a type II second-degree AV block.
- Has new onset bundle branch block related to an acute myocardial infarction.
- Has a bundle branch block with a first-degree AV block.
  - *QRS Complex:* Wide
  - *T Wave:* Tall and broad

11.15 How should the patient be treated before transcutaneous pacing?

The patient should be sedated if the patient is conscious because transcutaneous pacing is painful.

11.16 What would you expect a health care provider to do in an obese patient when performing transcutaneous pacing?

Higher milliamperes are required for the obese patients or those with large muscle mass.

11.17 Where are electrodes inserted for transvenous pacing?

Electrodes are placed through one of the following veins: internal jugular vein, subclavian vein, antecubital vein, or femoral vein.

11.18 How is a permanent pacemaker implanted?

A permanent pacemaker is implanted by an electrophysiologist in the electrophysiology lab (EP lab) under local anesthetic, conscious sedation, or both. A pulse generator is placed beneath the skin on the nondominant side of the patient.

11.19 What is the advantage of biventricular pacing?

Biventricular pacing reduces ventricular remodeling that can result from single ventricular pacing and can improve cardiac function in patients who have congestive heart failure. In biventricular pacing one electrode is inserted into the right ventricle against the septum and another electrode is inserted in the lateral wall of the left ventricle.

11.20 What is capture?

Capture is the impulse that causes the myocardium to contract.

11.21 What is capture threshold?

Capture threshold is the minimum milliamperes required to capture. A QRS complex is seen on an ECG after each pacing impulse.

11.22 What is failure to capture?

In failure to capture, the impulse fails to contract the myocardium. There is a pacing impulse without a QRS complex.

11.23 What are causes of failure to capture?

- Failure to capture can be caused by:
  - The impulse occurs during the absolute refractory period or the wrong point in the cardiac cycle.
  - High pacing thresholds caused by:
    - Acidosis/alkalosis
    - Hyperkalemia
    - Broken wires
    - Pacemaker box failure
    - Bad connection to an external pulse generator
    - Battery failure
    - An inflammatory reaction or fibrosis at the electrode-myocardium interface

11.24 What is failure to sense?

Failure to sense occurs when the pacemaker fails to sense intrinsic cardiac activity in demand pacing and is unable to deliver the impulse appropriately. Decreased milliamperes increase sensitivity to intrinsic activity. Conversely, increased milliamperes decrease sensitivity. The patient detects undersensing because the intrinsic activity is insufficient to provide cardiac output. The patient detects oversensing by experiencing additional impulses.

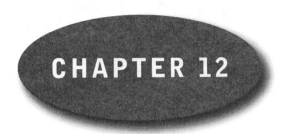

CHAPTER 12

Cardiac Instability

12.1   Definition

Cardiac instability occurs when cardiac output decreases sufficiently that the patient becomes hemodynamically unstable resulting in abnormal or unstable blood pressure. The patient becomes symptomatic as cardiac dysrhythmia occurs. Cardiac dysrhythmia has a profound effect on patients who have heart disease.

When confronted with a patient who becomes hemodynamically unstable, the health care provider must perform a thorough assessment in order to select treatment that reduces the risk of morbidity.

12.2   Acute Causes of Hemodynamic Instability

There are a number of conditions that can result in a patient becoming hemodynamically unstable. These are:

- **Hypovolemia:** Hypovolemia occurs when intravascular volume falls low enough to effect filling pressures. This is referred to as low filling pressure. Low filling pressure is measured by preload, central venous pressure (CVP), or left ventricular end diastolic pressure (LVEDP). Low filling pressure can be caused by:

    o Loss of blood from trauma or gastrointestinal (GI) bleeding

    o Dehydration from insufficient fluid intake or excessive fluid loss from diabetic ketoacidosis or excessive diarrhea or vomiting

- **Slow Heart Rate:** The heart rate is not fast enough to produce adequate blood pressure and perfusion of vital organs. As a result the cardiac output decreases, although the volume of blood ejected from the ventricles with each beat remains appropriately at 70 mL, which is a normal stroke volume. Cardiac output is the product of heart rate and stroke volume.

- **Fast Heart Rate:** The heart rate is too fast, therefore reducing the time for diastole, resulting in less filling time and a low stroke volume. Depending on the condition of the heart and the patient's health, this reduction in stroke volume may not be tolerated.

- **Pump Failure:** The heart has become an ineffective pump as a result of an acute myocardial infarction (AMI) or cardiomyopathy.

- *Acute Myocardial Infarction:* As a result of an AMI, portions of the myocardium cannot effectively contract because of injured or deadened cardiac tissue.

- *Cardiomyopathy:* Cardiomyopathy results in the inability of the heart to sufficiently pump blood. This causes a residual amount of blood to be retained in the left ventricle after systole. There are two types of cardiomyopathy:

  - Dilated Cardiomyopathy: The heart weakens and becomes enlarged.

  - Restricted Cardiomyopathy: The heart stiffens and prevents cardiac chambers to properly fill with blood.

12.3 Signs and Symptoms of Hemodynamic Instability

Clinical signs and symptoms of hemodynamic instability are:

- Altered Mental Status: Agitation or confusion

- Decreased Level of Consciousness: Lethargy or unresponsiveness

- Hemodynamics

  - Blood pressure, systolic less than 80 mm Hg; also, how symptomatic is the patient?

  - Cardiac index: 2.2 L/min/m^2 or less

- Diaphoretic

- Dizziness or lightheadedness

- Difficulty breathing or apneic

- No urine output or less than 0.5 mL/kg/hr caused by hypovolemia or kidneys not being perfused

- Chest pain

- Cardiac failure

12.4 Treatment of Hemodynamic Instability

The treatment for a hemodynamically unstable patient requires that the signs and symptoms of dysrhythmia be recognized early and emergency medical service, rapid response teams, or the code team be called immediately. Cardiopulmonary resuscitation, advanced cardiac life support, and timely defibrillation must be initiated if indicated.

Advanced cardiac life support treatment depends on the nature of the patient's condition. This can be:

- Bradycardia

- Tachycardia

- Atrial fibrillation and atrial flutter

- Pulseless ventricular fibrillation and ventricular tachycardia

- Asystole and pulseless electrical activity

12.5 Bradycardia

Bradycardia occurs when the patient's heart rate falls below 60 bpm. If the patient presents with sinus brady-cardia (normal rhythm with low heart rate) or bradycardia with third-degree AV block (irregular rhythm with low heart rate), then the following steps should be taken to return the patient to normal sinus rhythm:

- Administer atropine.

  - Atropine blocks the vagal response of the SA and AV nodes. The vagal response slows the heart rate. By blocking the vagal response, the SA and AV nodes are able to restore a normal heart rate.

  - Dose: 0.5 mg IV push every 3 to 5 minutes for a total dose of 0.03–0.04 mg/kg. Doses less than 0.5 mg can have a paradoxic slowing effect on the heart rate.

  - Caution:

    - Use in those patients in whom bradycardia may be a result of an acute coronary syndrome (ACS) or infarction. Speeding up the heart rate increases myocardial oxygen consumption, thus worsening the area of ischemia or infarct.

    - Atropine is not effective in infranodal blocks such as a second-degree type II with a wide QRS.

    - Not appropriate in patients who have undergone cardiac transplant, because of denervation where the vagus nerve is severed.

- Prepare for pacing:

  - Transcutaneous pacing (TCP) if the patient is not responding to atropine or there is a new-onset third-degree block related to ACS.

  - Transvenous pacing.

  - Pacing should begin immediately for patients who have severe symptoms from second- and third-degree blocks.

Bradycardia with Hypotension

Bradycardia with hypotension occurs when the patient's heart rate falls below 60 beats per minute and results in a decrease in blood pressure. Treat the patient by:

- Administering atropine (see section 12.5, Bradycardia)

- If this fails to establish a normal heart rate, then administer either:

  - Epinephrine 2 to 10 mcg/min titrated to heart rate, blood pressure, and systemic perfusion

  - Dopamine 5 to 10 mcg/kg/min titrated to heart rate, blood pressure, and systemic perfusion

- Administering fluids to correct hypovolemia

- Pacing

12.6   Tachycardia

Tachycardia occurs when the patient's heart rate is greater than 100 bpm. First assess:

- Is the patient stable or unstable?
  - Signs of an unstable patient:
    - Chest pains
    - Hypotension
    - Dizziness
    - Syncope
    - Pulmonary edema
- Are the symptoms related to pulmonary disease or cardiac disease?
- Is the QRS complex wide or narrow? A narrow complex QRS tachycardia may indicate:
  - Sinus tachycardia
  - Supraventricular tachycardia (SVT)
  - Atrial fibrillation
  - Atrial flutter

Wide complex tachycardia may indicate:

- Ventricular tachycardia
- Supraventricular tachycardia
  - Is the rhythm regular or irregular?

Sinus Tachycardia

Sinus tachycardia is a normal sinus rhythm with a heart rate of greater than 100 bpm. Identify and treat the underlying cause of sinus tachycardia. Common causes of sinus tachycardia are:

- Fever
- Pain
- Anxiety
- Infection
- Hyperthyroid
- Exercise
- Anemia

Stable and Unstable Supraventricular Tachycardia

Supraventricular tachycardia is a tachycardic rhythm that originates above the ventricles. Patients can present with either a narrow or wide QRS complex. Treatment methods depend on whether the patient is stable or unstable. A stable patient shows no obvious signs or symptoms. An unstable patient shows signs or symptoms.

Stable Patient

- **Vagal Maneuver:** Ask the patient to bear down as if having a bowel movement. This causes a vagal response that slows the heart rate.
- **Administer Adenosine:**
  - First dose = 6 mg IV rapid push followed with a 20 mL normal saline flush.
  - Second dose = 12 mg IV rapid push followed by a 20 mL normal saline flush.
  - Third dose = 12 mg IV rapid push followed by a 20 mL normal saline flush.
  - If not effective after the third dose, adenosine will most likely not work.
  - May slow the rhythm enough to reveal flutter waves or atrial fibrillation (diagnostic of these two rhythms).

Unstable Patient

- Administer one round of adenosine (see Stable Patient).
- Administer synchronized cardioversion if adenosine does not restore normal sinus rhythm.
- If synchronized cardioversion fails (see Unstable Pulseless SVT with Wide QRS Complex).

12.7   Atrial Fibrillation and Atrial Flutter

If the patient presents with atrial fibrillation or atrial flutter, assess whether the patient is stable (no signs or symptoms) or unstable (patient is symptomatic). The treatment method depends on the stability of the patient.

Stable Patient

- Control the heart rate with medication.
  - The goal is to re-establish a heart rate of less than 100 bpm. This is accomplished by administering:
    - Calcium channel blockers
      - Diltiazem 10 to 20 mg IV depending on weight, administer the bolus over 2 minutes followed by a 5 to 15 mg/hour maintenance infusion
      - Verapamil 5 to 10 mg IV over 2 minutes; may repeat in 30 minutes
    - Beta blockers
      - Propranolol 1 mg IV over 2 minutes; may repeat every 5 minutes to a maximum of 5 mg
        - 1 to 3 mg IV every 4 hours

- Digoxin
  - 0.25 to 0.5 mg IV; then 0.25 mg IV every 4 to 6 hours to maximum of 1 mg in a 24hr period
  - 0.125 to 0.25 mg per day IV or orally
- Convert the rhythm with medication.
  - The goal is to re-establish a normal sinus rhythm. This is accomplished by administering the following medications. The dose depends on the patient's renal and hepatic function, co-morbidities, drug interactions and overall cardiac function.
    - Quinidine
    - Cordarone (if ejection fraction is less than 35%)
    - Flecainide
    - Ibutilide
    - Dofetilide
  - Administer a transesophageal echocardiogram to assess if blood clots exist in the atria.
    - If no clots are present and the patient is administered IV anticoagulation, then perform a cardioversion.
- Administer IV anticoagulation to prevent blood clots.
  - Administer if the condition of atrial fibrillation has been longer than 48 hours, especially if considering cardioversion in the future.
  - Patient should be therapeutic on warfarin for at least 3 weeks before cardioversion and 4 weeks after cardioversion.
  - Monitor INR closely if on Cordarone and warfarin simultaneously; INR may be abnormally high.

Unstable Patient

Perform synchronized cardioversion. Administer sedation if the patient is conscious. The cardioversion settings depend on whether the biphasic or monophasic unit is being used.

- Biphasic 100J to 120J
- Monophasic
  - First shock 100J to 200J
  - Second shock 300J
  - Third shock 360J

12.8   Pulseless Ventricular Fibrillation/Ventricular Tachycardia

A pulseless ventricular fibrillation occurs when the ventricles quiver rather than contract properly and no pulse is detected. Ventricular tachycardia occurs when the ventricles contract very quickly, greater than 180 bpm. Both conditions can lead to sudden death. These conditions should be treated the following way.

- Cardiopulmonary resuscitation (CPR).
  - If the patient is a witnessed collapse notify EMS immediately.

- o If time of arrest is unknown perform CPR for 2 minutes. Do not interrupt CPR except for defibrillating. Then notify EMS.

- o Maintain continuous chest compressions with little to no interruptions.

- Defibrillate or use automated external defibrillator (AED) if the patient is not responding to CPR.

  - o Biphasic: 120J to 200J.

  - o Monophasic: 360J.

  - o One shock and resume CPR for 2 minutes; there is a better chance of survival with continued CPR rather than stacked shocks.

- Administer medication.

  - o Vasopressors increase myocardial and cerebral blood flow and increase aortic diastolic pressure and coronary perfusion pressure. Administer either epinephrine or vasopressin.

    - ▪ Epinephrine:

      - ♦ Increases the heart rate

      - ♦ Increases systolic and diastolic blood pressure

      - ♦ Increases myocardial oxygen consumption

      - ♦ Increases coronary and cerebral blood flow

      - ♦ Dose: 1 mg IV/IO every 3 to 5 minutes; no limit on how much can be given

      - ♦ May be given 3 to 5 minutes after a dose of vasopressin if additional vasopressors are needed

    - ▪ Vasopressin:

      - ♦ Does not increase myocardial oxygen consumption because vasopressin does not have beta-adrenergic activity.

      - ♦ Dose: 40 U IV/IO to replace the first or second dose of epinephrine

- Administer antiarrhythmics to suppress fast cardiac rhythms. Amiodarone and lidocaine should not be administered together. Administer only one of these medications.

  - o Amiodarone:

    - ▪ Initial dose: 300 mg IV/IO

    - ▪ Subsequent dose: An additional dose of 150 mg IV/IO in 3 to 5 minutes

  - o Lidocaine:

    - ▪ Initial Dose: 1 to 1.5 mg/kg IV push

    - ▪ Subsequent Dose: 0.5 mg to 0.75 mg/kg IV every 3 to 5 minutes

    - ▪ Maximum Dose: 3 mg/kg

- Administer magnesium to terminate polymorphic ventricular tachycardia with prolonged QT interval:

  - o Dose: 1 to 2 g diluted in 10 mL D5W IV push over 10 minutes

12.9 Asystole and Pulseless Electrical Activity (PEA)

Asystole is a state in which there is no ECG wave; this is commonly known as *flat line*. The patient has insufficient electrical activity to produce any pulse.

Pulseless electrical activity (PEA) occurs when the patient does not have a pulse. This can be caused by a number of underlying conditions. The patient's pulse is re-established once the underlying condition is corrected. These conditions are:

- Hypovolemia

- Hypoxia

- Acidosis

- Hyperkalemia/hypokalemia

- Hypoglycemia

- Hypothermia

- Drug overdoses

- Tamponade

- Tension pneumothorax

- Thrombosis

- Trauma

A patient who is asystole or PEA should be treated with CPR; do not defibrillate or use an automated external defibrillator (AED). Defibrillation causes the heart to stop beating for a moment sufficient for the patient's natural cardiac pacemaker (SA node) to re-establish a normal sinus rhythm. However, in asystole and PEA, the patient does not have a heart contraction and therefore there is no reason to defibrillate the patient.

Also administer:

- Vasopressors (see section 12.8, Pulseless Ventricular Fibrillation/Ventricular Tachycardia)

- Atropine (see section 12.5, Bradycardia)

  ○ Dose: 1 mg every 3 minutes until reaching a maximum dose of 0.04 mg/kg

- Sodium bicarbonate

  ○ To reverse hyperkalemia and the possible tricyclic antidepressant overdose that may have caused this condition

  ○ Dose: 1 mEq/kg

Solved Problems

Cardiac Instability

12.1   When does cardiac instability occur?

Cardiac instability occurs when cardiac output decreases sufficiently that the patient becomes hemodynamically unstable.

12.2   What is hemodynamically unstable?

Hemodynamically unstable means there is abnormal or unstable blood pressure. The patient becomes symptomatic as cardiac dysrhythmia occurs.

12.3   What should you do if the patient is hemodynamically unstable?

When confronted with a patient who becomes hemodynamically unstable, the health care provider must perform a thorough assessment to select treatment that reduces the risk of morbidity.

12.4   What is hypovolemia?

Hypovolemia occurs when blood pressure falls below a pressure level within the circulatory system to adequately fill blood vessels with blood.

12.5   What is low filling pressure?

Low filling pressure means that a patient is hypovolemic.

12.6   How is filling pressure measured?

Filling pressure is measured by preload, central venous pressure (CVP), or left ventricular end diastolic pressure (LVEDP).

12.7   What can cause hypovolemia?

- Losses of blood from trauma or gastroin tetinal bleeding

- Dehydration from insufficient fluid intake, excessive fluid loss from diabetic ketoacidosis, or excessive diarrhea or vomiting

12.8   How can a slow heart rate cause a patient to become hemodynamically unstable?

The heart rate is not enough to produce adequate blood pressure and perfusion of vital organs.

12.9   How can a fast heart rate cause a patient to become hemodynamically unstable?

The heart rate is too fast, therefore reducing the time for diastole resulting in less filling time and a low stroke volume depending on the condition of the heart and the patient's health.

12.10   What are symptoms of a hemodynamically unstable patient?

- Altered mental status: agitation or confusion

- Decreased level of consciousness: lethargy or unresponsiveness

- Hemodynamics

  o Blood pressure: Systolic less than 80 mm Hg; Also, how symptomatic is the patient?

  o Cardiac index: 2.2 $L/min/m^2$ or less

- Diaphoretic

- Dizziness or lightheadedness

- Difficulty breathing or apneic

- No urine output caused by hypovolemia or kidneys not being perfused

- Chest pain

- Cardiac failure

12.11 Why is atropine administered to a patient who has bradycardia?

Atropine blocks the vagal response of the SA and AV nodes. The vagal response slows the heart rate. By blocking the vagal response, the SA and AV node are able to restore a normal heart rate.

12.12 Why is atropine not effective in patients who have undergone cardiac transplants?

The patient has undergone denervation where the vagus nerve is severed.

12.13 What should be done if the patient does not respond to atropine?

Transcutaneous pacing is used as a temporary solution to maintaining a sinus rhythm until either transvenous pacing is implemented or an internal permanent pacemaker is implanted into the patient.

12.14 If a patient has bradycardia and hypotension, what should be done if atropine fails to re-establish a normal heart rate?

If this fails to establish a normal heart rate, then administer either:

- Epinephrine 2 to 10 mcg/min titrated to heart rate, blood pressure, and systemic perfusion
- Dopamine 2 to 10 mcg/min titrated to heart rate, blood pressure, and systemic perfusion

12.15 What are the signs of an unstable patient who has tachycardia?

The signs of an unstable patient are chest pains, hypotension, dizziness, syncope, and pulmonary edema.

12.16 What might be the underlying cause of narrow complex QRS tachycardia?

The possible underlying causes of narrow complex QRS tachycardia are sinus tachycardia, supraventricular tachycardia, atrial fibrillation, and atrial flutter.

12.17 What might be the causes of sinus tachycardia?

The possible underlying causes of sinus tachycardia are fever, pain, anxiety, infection, hyperthyroid, exercise, and anemia.

12.18 What would be the first treatment for a stable patient who has supraventricular tachycardia?

The first treatment for a stable patient who has supraventricular tachycardia is a vagal maneuver. Ask the patient to bear down as if having a bowel movement. This causes a vagal response that slows the heart rate.

12.19 What is supraventricular tachycardia?

Supraventricular tachycardia is a tachycardic rhythm that originates above the ventricles.

12.20 What are the three treatment methods for a patient who is diagnosed with atrial flutter?

Control the heart rate. Control the heart rhythm. Prevent blood clots from forming.

12.21 How do you know if a patient with atrial flutter has blood clots in the atria?

Administer a transesophageal echocardiography to assess if blood clots exist in the atria.

12.22 Why would blood clots form in the atria if the patient has atrial flutter?

There is a risk that blood will pool and not circulate. Pooling blood is susceptible to blood clots.

12.23 What should be performed if the patient who has atrial flutter becomes unstable?

If the patient who has atrial flutter becomes unstable, perform synchronized cardioversion.

12.24 What is the rationale for administering vasopressors?

Vasopressors increase myocardial and cerebral blood flow.

12.25 Why might a health care provider administer vasopressin instead of epinephrine?

Vasopressin does not increase myocardial oxygen consumption. Vasopressin does not have beta-adrenergic activity. Epinephrine increases myocardial oxygen consumption, which may be disadvantageous to the patient.

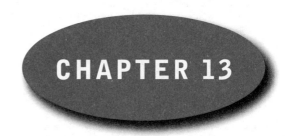

CHAPTER 13

Practice Strips

Fill in the blanks under the following practice strips to test your ability to interpret ECGs for cardiac rhythm (strips 13.1–13.114) and cardiac pacing (strips 13.115–13.131). Answers are provided on pages 237–247.

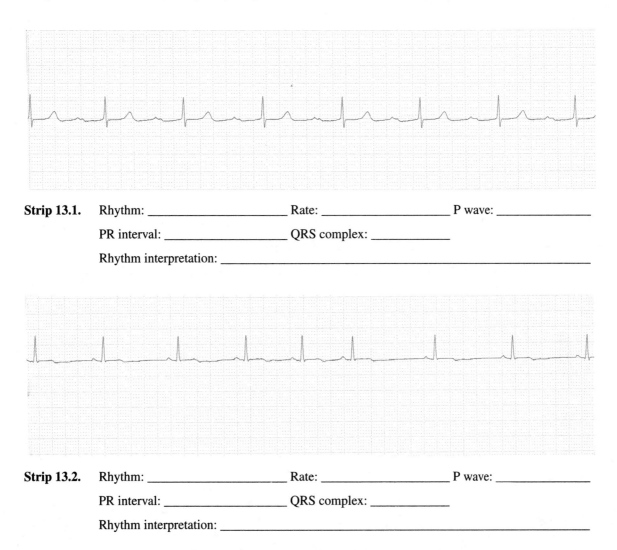

Strip 13.1.   Rhythm: _____ Rate: _____ P wave: _____

PR interval: _____ QRS complex: _____

Rhythm interpretation: _____

Strip 13.2.   Rhythm: _____ Rate: _____ P wave: _____

PR interval: _____ QRS complex: _____

Rhythm interpretation: _____

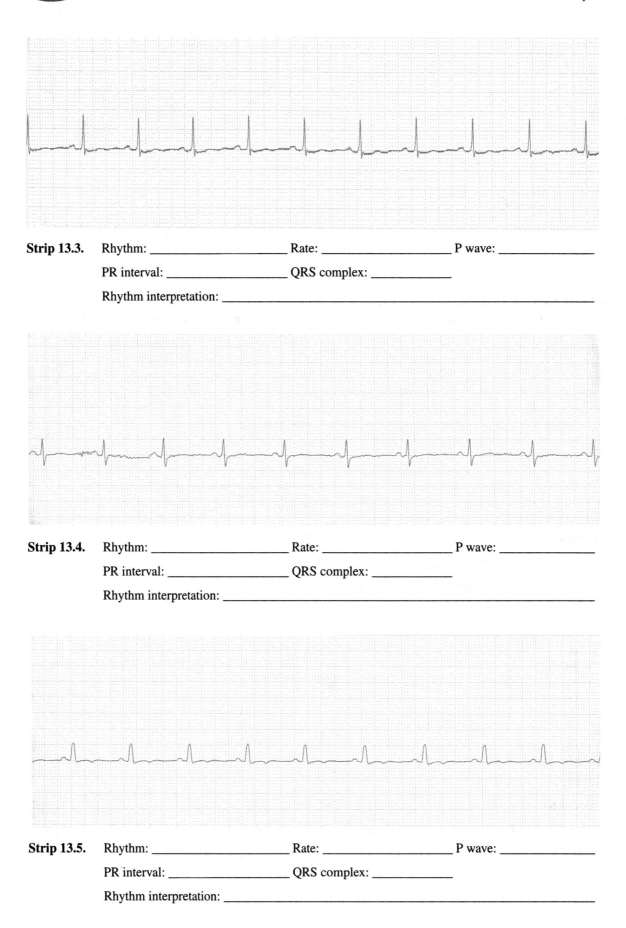

Strip 13.3. Rhythm: _____ Rate: _____ P wave: _____

PR interval: _____ QRS complex: _____

Rhythm interpretation: _____

Strip 13.4. Rhythm: _____ Rate: _____ P wave: _____

PR interval: _____ QRS complex: _____

Rhythm interpretation: _____

Strip 13.5. Rhythm: _____ Rate: _____ P wave: _____

PR interval: _____ QRS complex: _____

Rhythm interpretation: _____

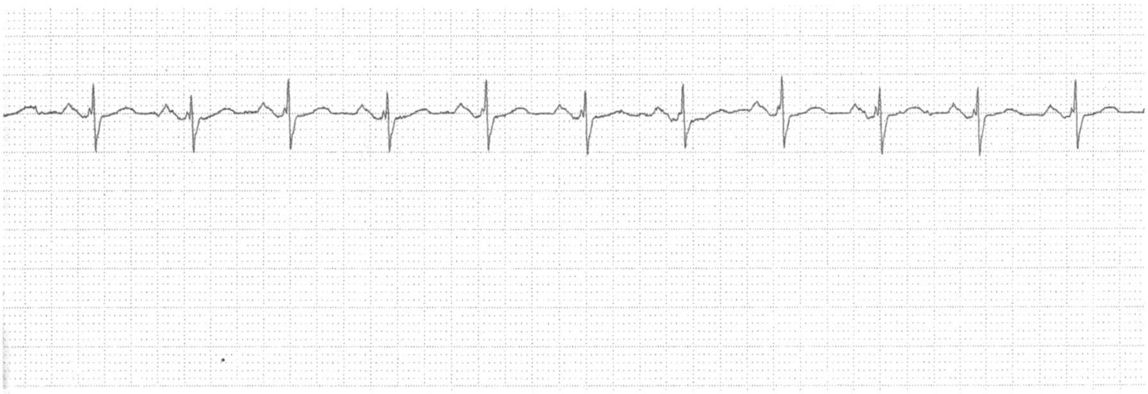

Strip 13.6.   Rhythm: _____ Rate: _____ P wave: _____

PR interval: _____ QRS complex: _____

Rhythm interpretation: _____

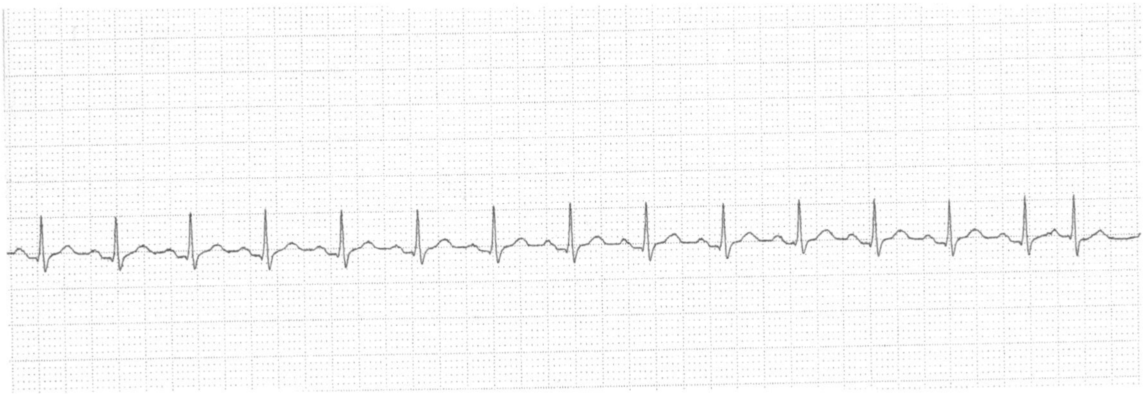

Strip 13.7.   Rhythm: _____ Rate: _____ P wave: _____

PR interval: _____ QRS complex: _____

Rhythm interpretation: _____

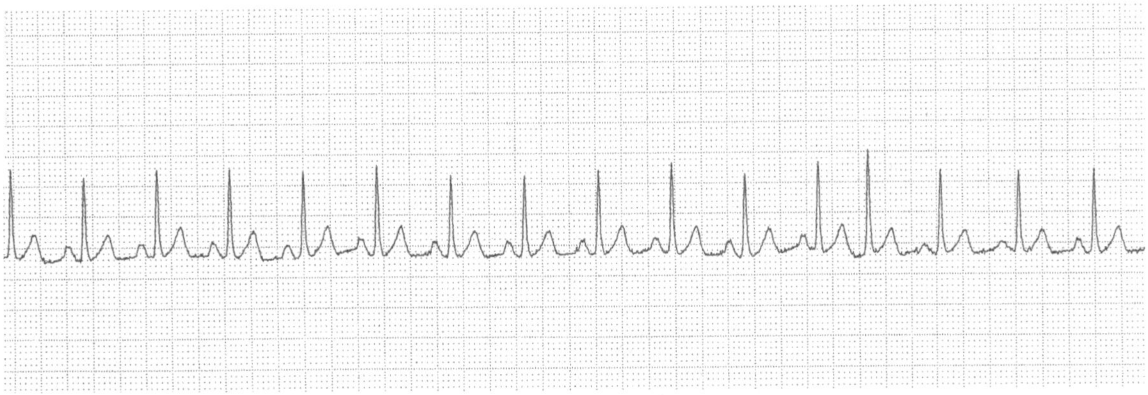

Strip 13.8.   Rhythm: _____ Rate: _____ P wave: _____

PR interval: _____ QRS complex: _____

Rhythm interpretation: _____

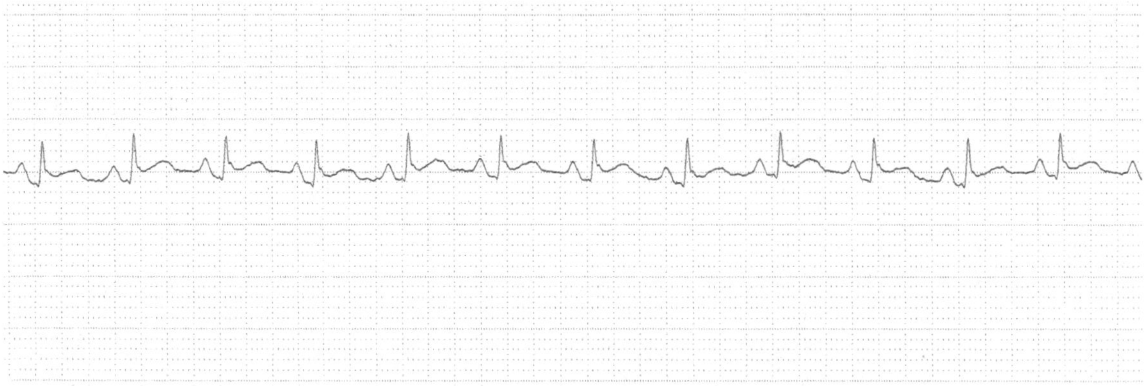

Strip 13.9. Rhythm: _____ Rate: _____ P wave: _____

PR interval: _____ QRS complex: _____

Rhythm interpretation: _____

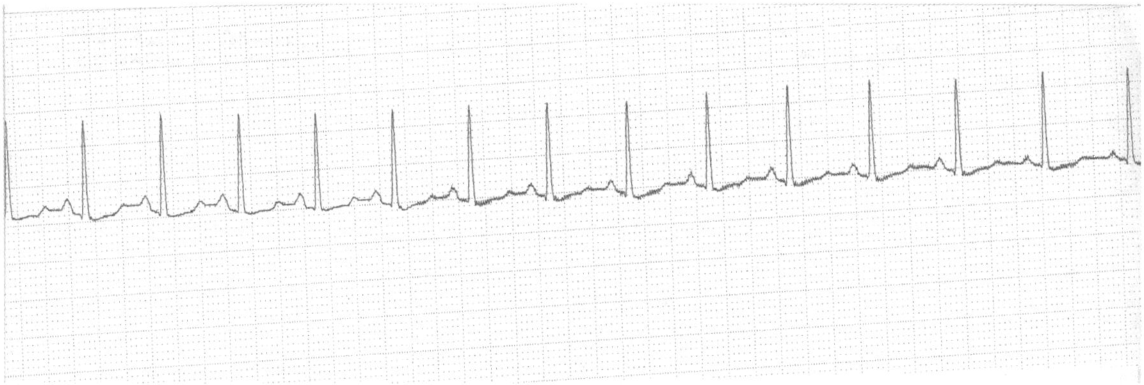

Strip 13.10. Rhythm: _____ Rate: _____ P wave: _____

PR interval: _____ QRS complex: _____

Rhythm interpretation: _____

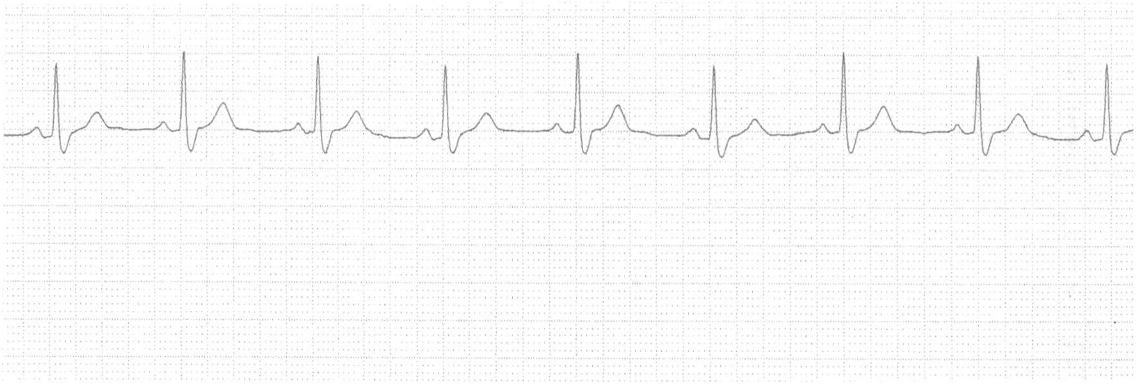

Strip 13.11. Rhythm: _____ Rate: _____ P wave: _____

PR interval: _____ QRS complex: _____

Rhythm interpretation: _____

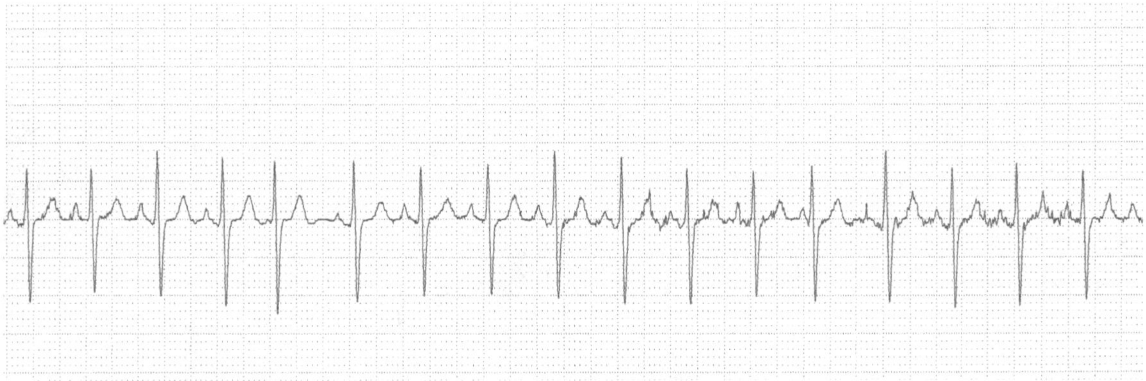

Strip 13.12. Rhythm: _____ Rate: _____ P wave: _____

PR interval: _____ QRS complex: _____

Rhythm interpretation: _____

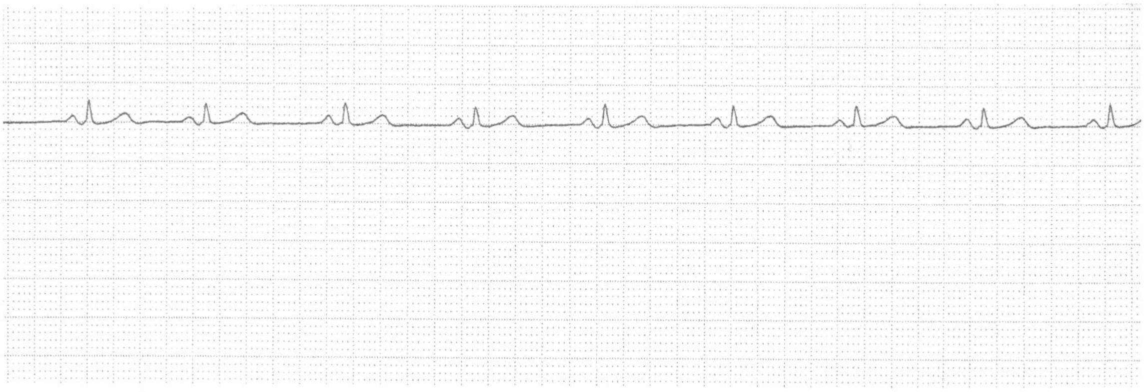

Strip 13.13. Rhythm: _____ Rate: _____ P wave: _____

PR interval: _____ QRS complex: _____

Rhythm interpretation: _____

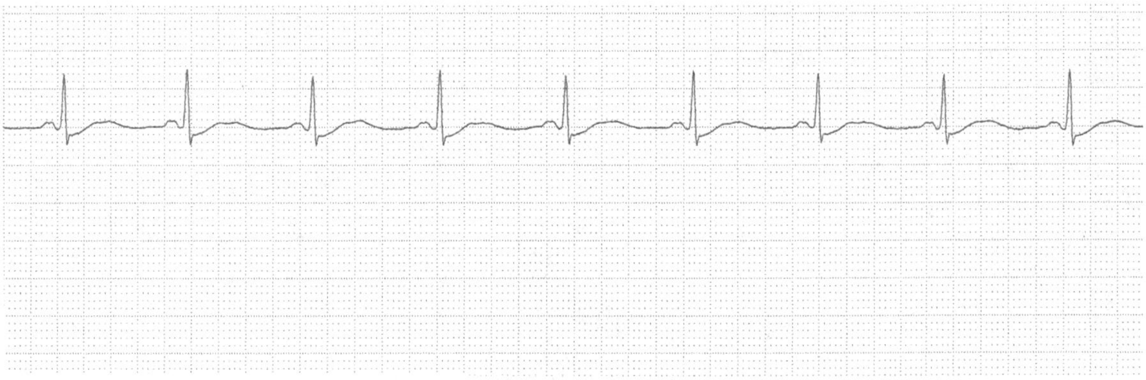

Strip 13.14. Rhythm: _____ Rate: _____ P wave: _____

PR interval: _____ QRS complex: _____

Rhythm interpretation: _____

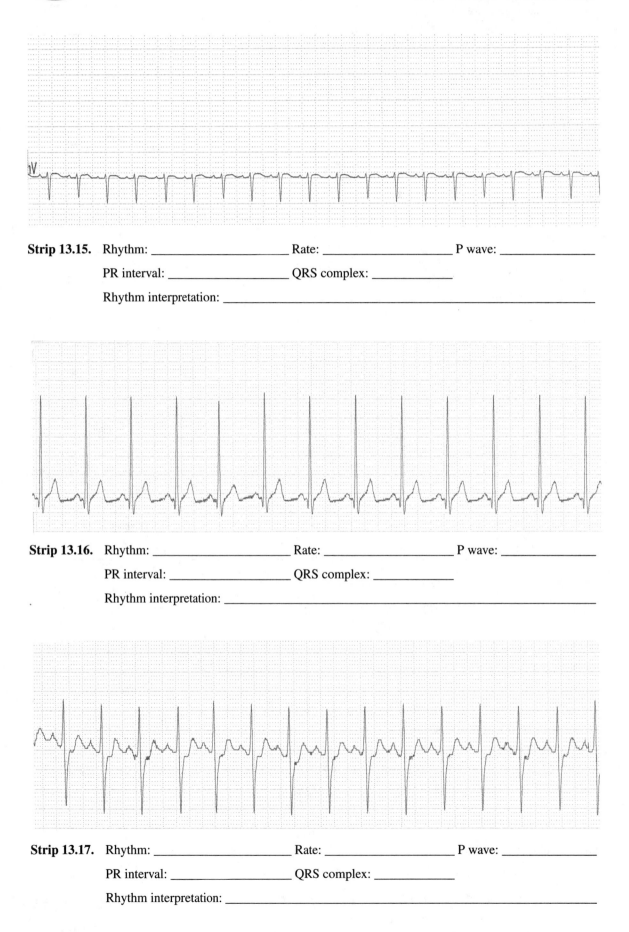

Strip 13.15. Rhythm: _____ Rate: _____ P wave: _____

PR interval: _____ QRS complex: _____

Rhythm interpretation: _____

Strip 13.16. Rhythm: _____ Rate: _____ P wave: _____

PR interval: _____ QRS complex: _____

Rhythm interpretation: _____

Strip 13.17. Rhythm: _____ Rate: _____ P wave: _____

PR interval: _____ QRS complex: _____

Rhythm interpretation: _____

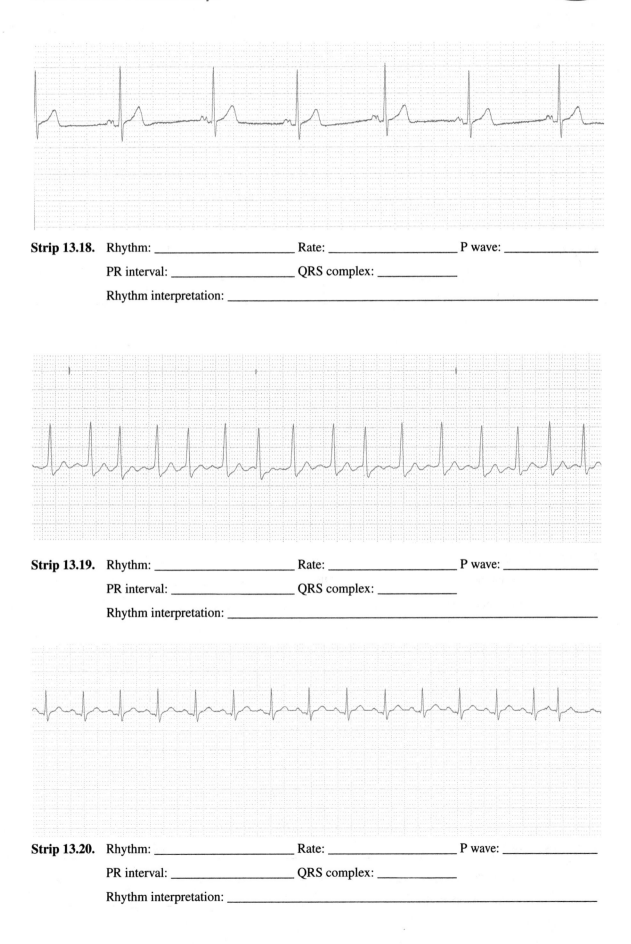

Strip 13.18. Rhythm: _____ Rate: _____ P wave: _____

PR interval: _____ QRS complex: _____

Rhythm interpretation: _____

Strip 13.19. Rhythm: _____ Rate: _____ P wave: _____

PR interval: _____ QRS complex: _____

Rhythm interpretation: _____

Strip 13.20. Rhythm: _____ Rate: _____ P wave: _____

PR interval: _____ QRS complex: _____

Rhythm interpretation: _____

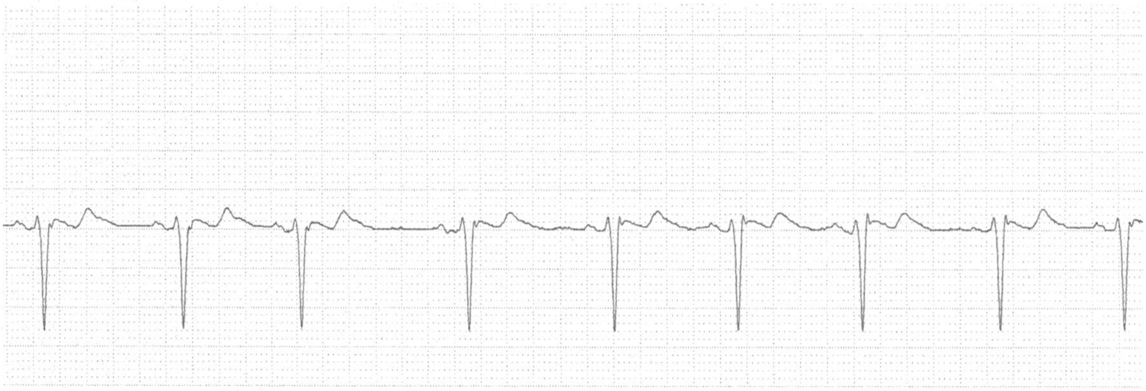

Strip 13.21. Rhythm: _____ Rate: _____ P wave: _____

PR interval: _____ QRS complex: _____

Rhythm interpretation: _____

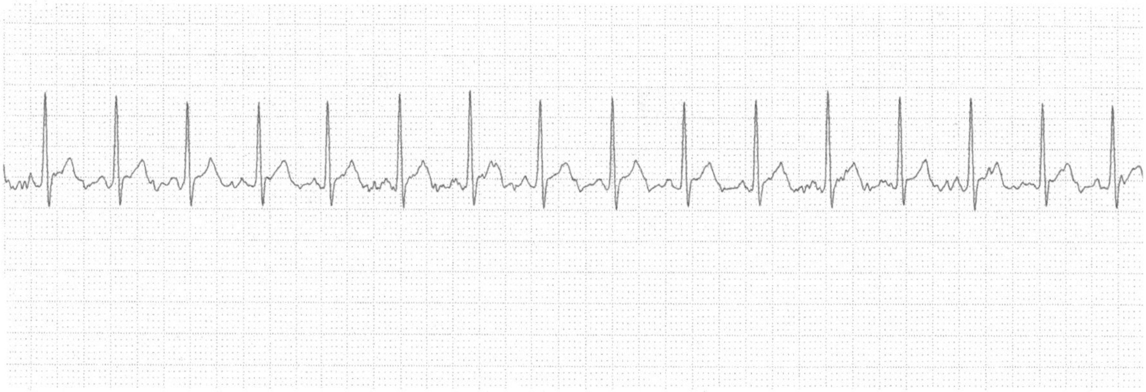

Strip 13.22. Rhythm: _____ Rate: _____ P wave: _____

PR interval: _____ QRS complex: _____

Rhythm interpretation: _____

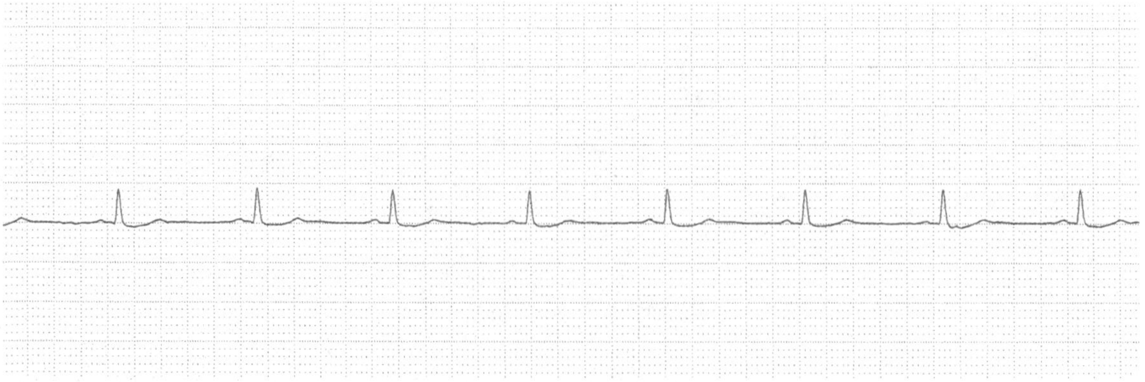

Strip 13.23. Rhythm: _____ Rate: _____ P wave: _____

PR interval: _____ QRS complex: _____

Rhythm interpretation: _____

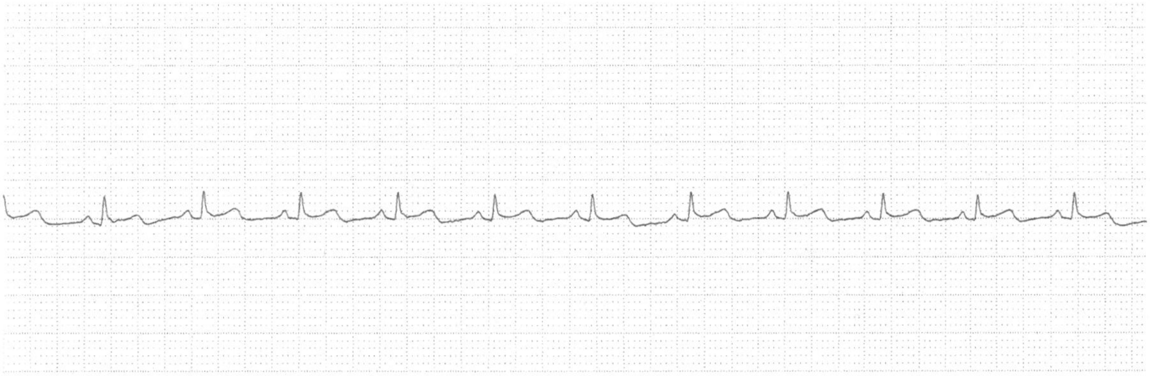

Strip 13.24. Rhythm: _____ Rate: _____ P wave: _____

PR interval: _____ QRS complex: _____

Rhythm interpretation: _____

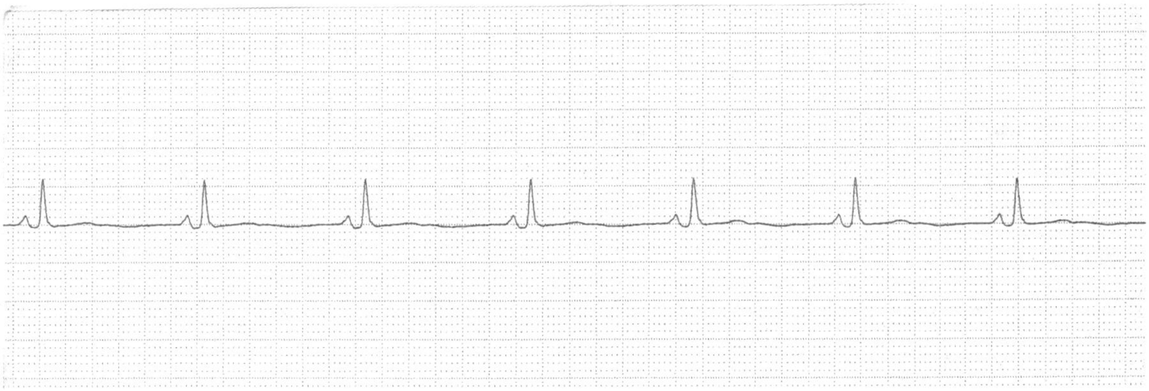

Strip 13.25. Rhythm: _____ Rate: _____ P wave: _____

PR interval: _____ QRS complex: _____

Rhythm interpretation: _____

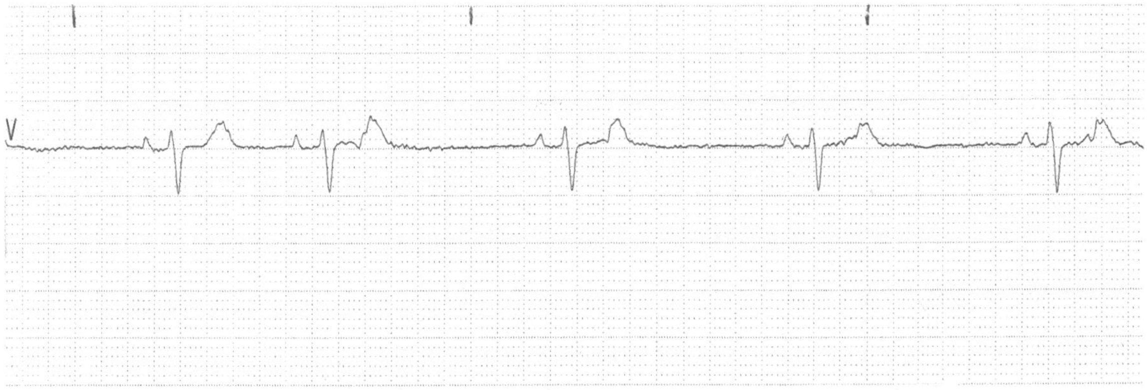

Strip 13.26. Rhythm: _____ Rate: _____ P wave: _____

PR interval: _____ QRS complex: _____

Rhythm interpretation: _____

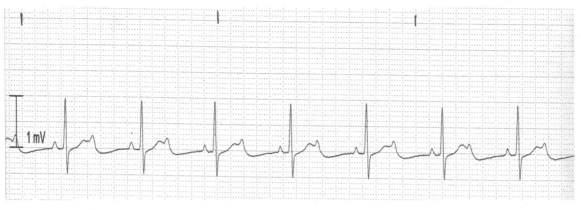

Strip 13.27. Rhythm: _____ Rate: _____ P wave: _____

PR interval: _____ QRS complex: _____

Rhythm interpretation: _____

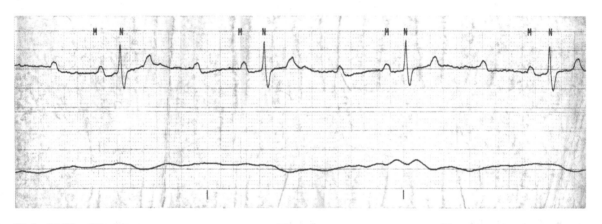

Strip 13.28. Rhythm: _____ Rate: _____ P wave: _____

PR interval: _____ QRS complex: _____

Rhythm interpretation: _____

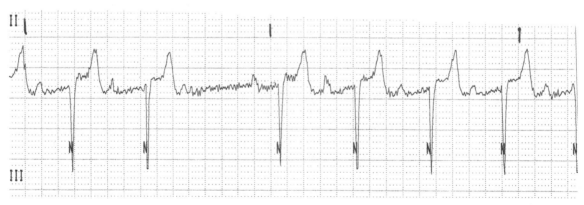

Strip 13.29. Rhythm: _____ Rate: _____ P wave: _____

PR interval: _____ QRS complex: _____

Rhythm interpretation: _____

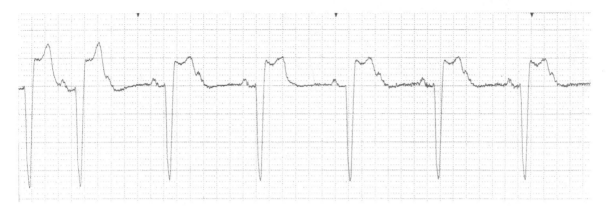

Strip 13.30. Rhythm: _____ Rate: _____ P wave: _____

PR interval: _____ QRS complex: _____

Rhythm interpretation: _____

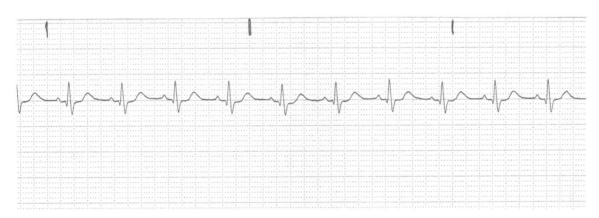

Strip 13.31. Rhythm: _____ Rate: _____ P wave: _____

PR interval: _____ QRS complex: _____

Rhythm interpretation: _____

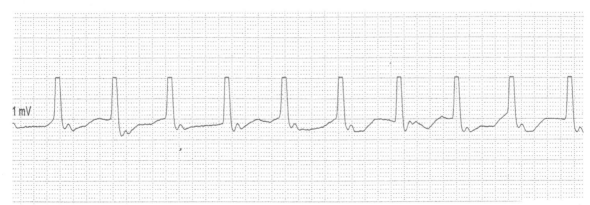

Strip 13.32. Rhythm: _____ Rate: _____ P wave: _____

PR interval: _____ QRS complex: _____

Rhythm interpretation: _____

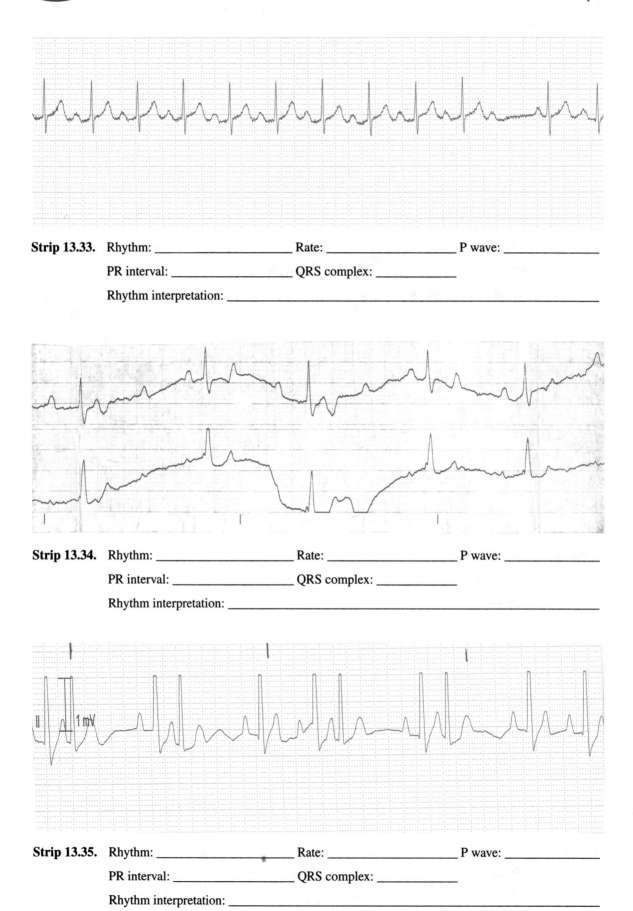

Strip 13.33. Rhythm: _____ Rate: _____ P wave: _____

PR interval: _____ QRS complex: _____

Rhythm interpretation: _____

Strip 13.34. Rhythm: _____ Rate: _____ P wave: _____

PR interval: _____ QRS complex: _____

Rhythm interpretation: _____

Strip 13.35. Rhythm: _____ Rate: _____ P wave: _____

PR interval: _____ QRS complex: _____

Rhythm interpretation: _____

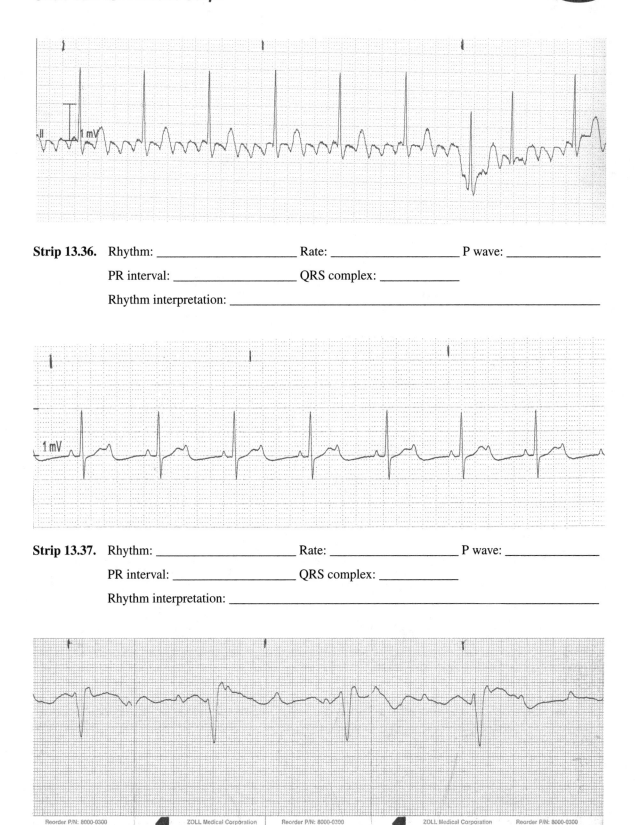

Strip 13.36. Rhythm: _____ Rate: _____ P wave: _____

PR interval: _____ QRS complex: _____

Rhythm interpretation: _____

Strip 13.37. Rhythm: _____ Rate: _____ P wave: _____

PR interval: _____ QRS complex: _____

Rhythm interpretation: _____

Strip 13.38. Rhythm: _____ Rate: _____ P wave: _____

PR interval: _____ QRS complex: _____

Rhythm interpretation: _____

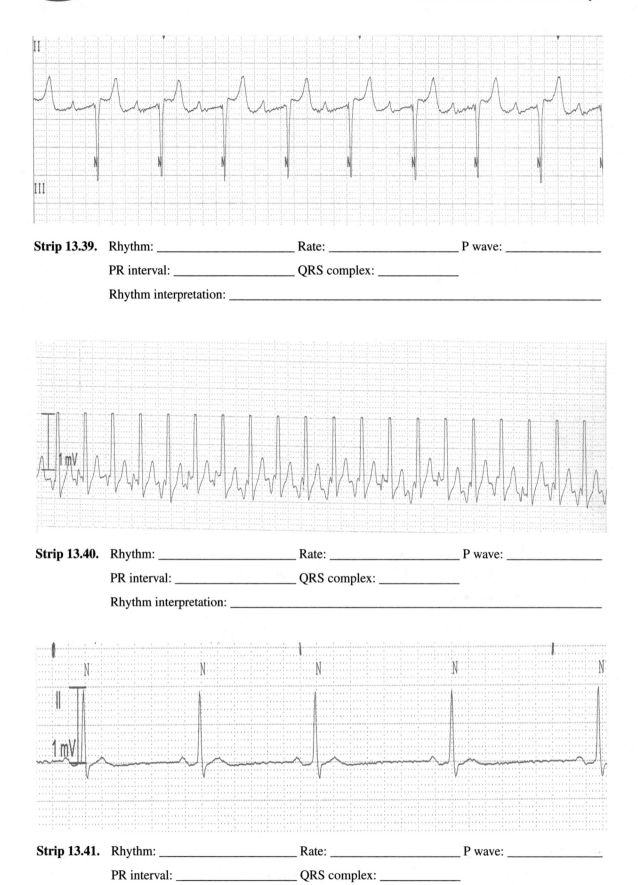

Strip 13.39. Rhythm: _____ Rate: _____ P wave: _____

PR interval: _____ QRS complex: _____

Rhythm interpretation: _____

Strip 13.40. Rhythm: _____ Rate: _____ P wave: _____

PR interval: _____ QRS complex: _____

Rhythm interpretation: _____

Strip 13.41. Rhythm: _____ Rate: _____ P wave: _____

PR interval: _____ QRS complex: _____

Rhythm interpretation: _____

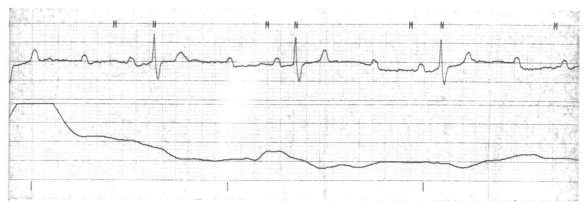

Strip 13.42. Rhythm: _____ Rate: _____ P wave: _____

PR interval: _____ QRS complex: _____

Rhythm interpretation: _____

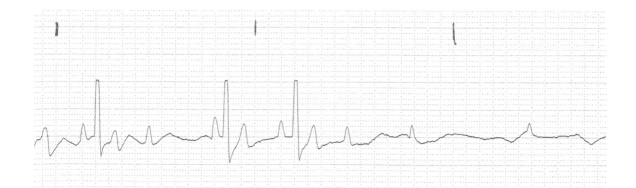

Strip 13.43. Rhythm: _____ Rate: _____ P wave: _____

PR interval: _____ QRS complex: _____

Rhythm interpretation: _____

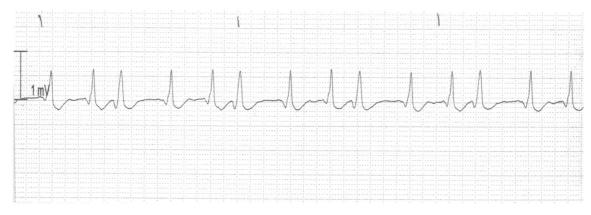

Strip 13.44. Rhythm: _____ Rate: _____ P wave: _____

PR interval: _____ QRS complex: _____

Rhythm interpretation: _____

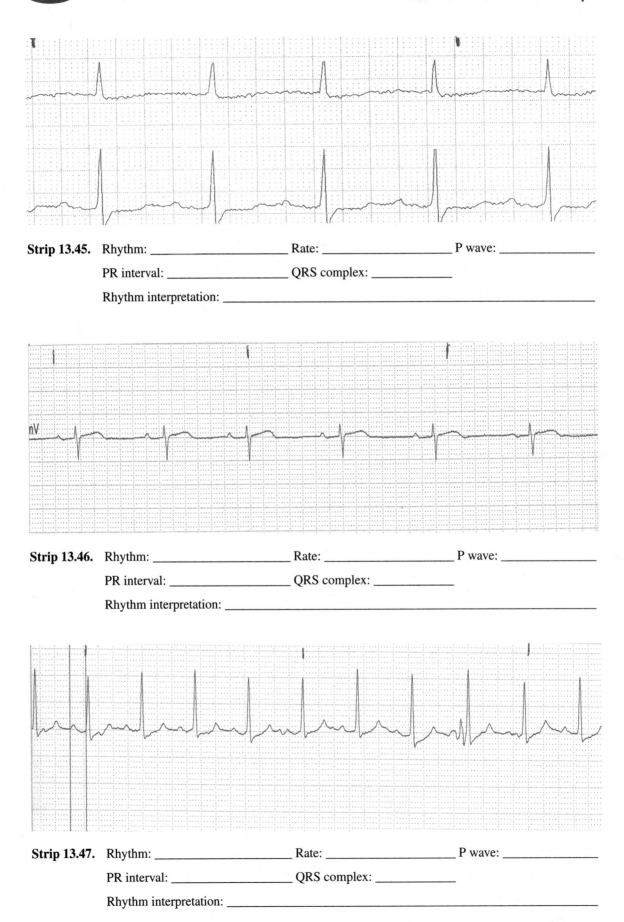

Strip 13.45. Rhythm: _____ Rate: _____ P wave: _____

PR interval: _____ QRS complex: _____

Rhythm interpretation: _____

Strip 13.46. Rhythm: _____ Rate: _____ P wave: _____

PR interval: _____ QRS complex: _____

Rhythm interpretation: _____

Strip 13.47. Rhythm: _____ Rate: _____ P wave: _____

PR interval: _____ QRS complex: _____

Rhythm interpretation: _____

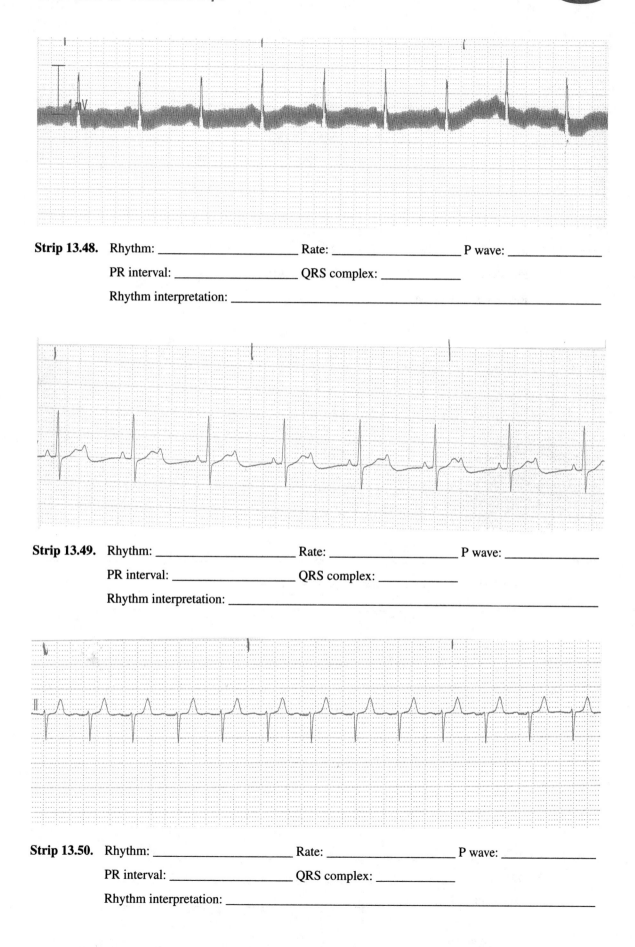

Strip 13.48. Rhythm: _____ Rate: _____ P wave: _____

PR interval: _____ QRS complex: _____

Rhythm interpretation: _____

Strip 13.49. Rhythm: _____ Rate: _____ P wave: _____

PR interval: _____ QRS complex: _____

Rhythm interpretation: _____

Strip 13.50. Rhythm: _____ Rate: _____ P wave: _____

PR interval: _____ QRS complex: _____

Rhythm interpretation: _____

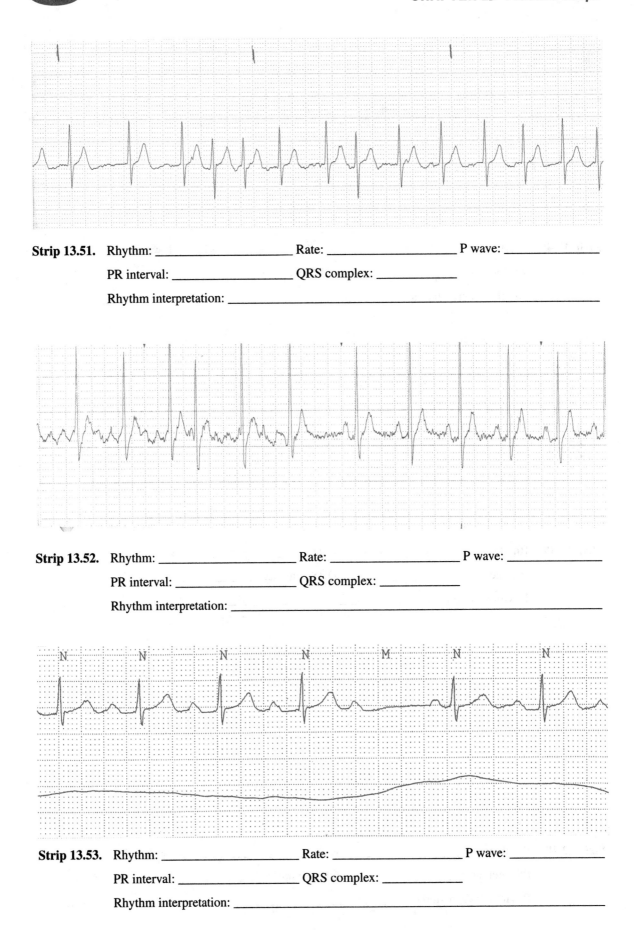

Strip 13.51. Rhythm: _____ Rate: _____ P wave: _____

PR interval: _____ QRS complex: _____

Rhythm interpretation: _____

Strip 13.52. Rhythm: _____ Rate: _____ P wave: _____

PR interval: _____ QRS complex: _____

Rhythm interpretation: _____

Strip 13.53. Rhythm: _____ Rate: _____ P wave: _____

PR interval: _____ QRS complex: _____

Rhythm interpretation: _____

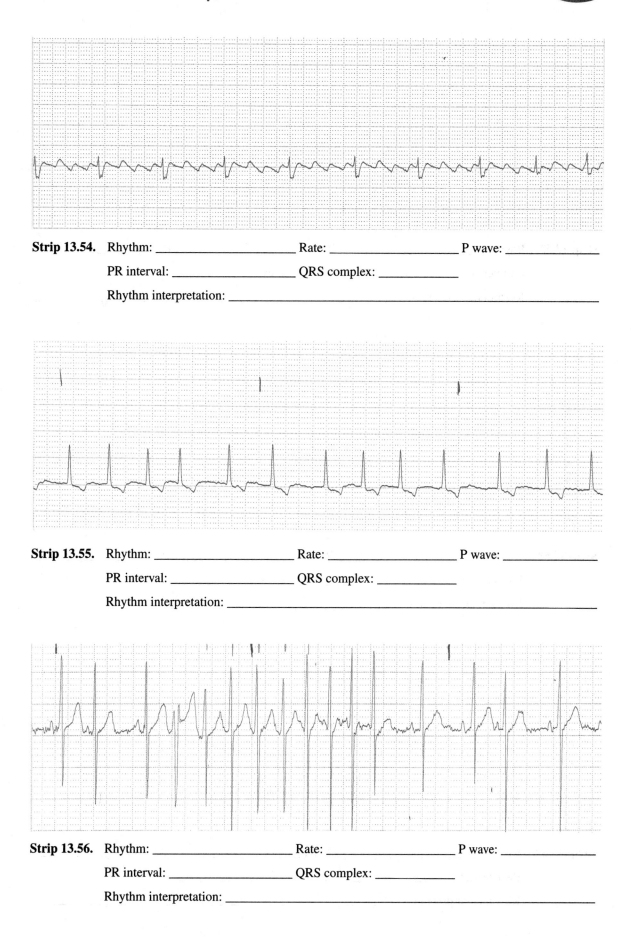

Strip 13.54. Rhythm: _____ Rate: _____ P wave: _____

PR interval: _____ QRS complex: _____

Rhythm interpretation: _____

Strip 13.55. Rhythm: _____ Rate: _____ P wave: _____

PR interval: _____ QRS complex: _____

Rhythm interpretation: _____

Strip 13.56. Rhythm: _____ Rate: _____ P wave: _____

PR interval: _____ QRS complex: _____

Rhythm interpretation: _____

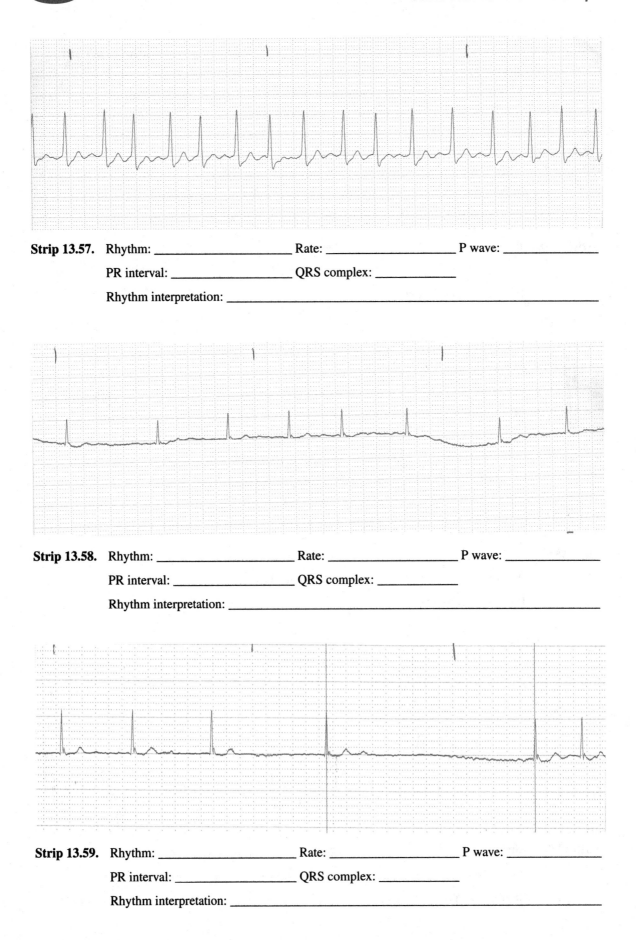

Strip 13.57. Rhythm: _____ Rate: _____ P wave: _____

PR interval: _____ QRS complex: _____

Rhythm interpretation: _____

Strip 13.58. Rhythm: _____ Rate: _____ P wave: _____

PR interval: _____ QRS complex: _____

Rhythm interpretation: _____

Strip 13.59. Rhythm: _____ Rate: _____ P wave: _____

PR interval: _____ QRS complex: _____

Rhythm interpretation: _____

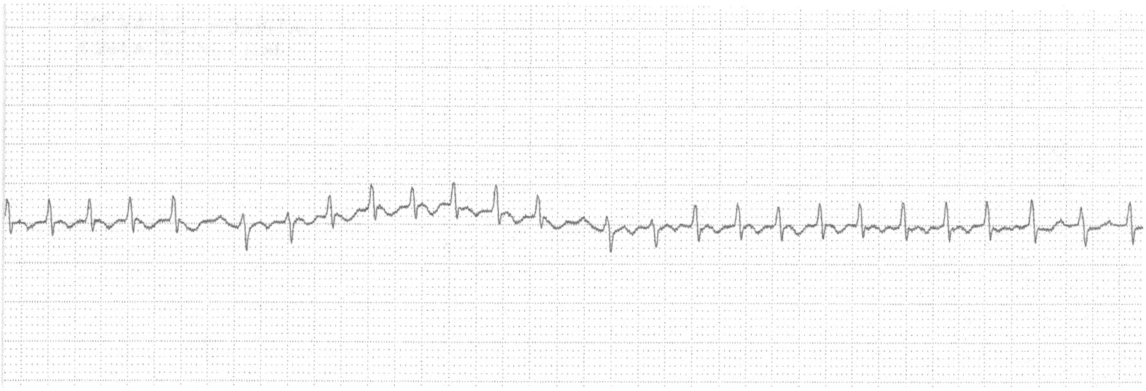

Strip 13.60. Rhythm: _____ Rate: _____ P wave: _____

PR interval: _____ QRS complex: _____

Rhythm interpretation: _____

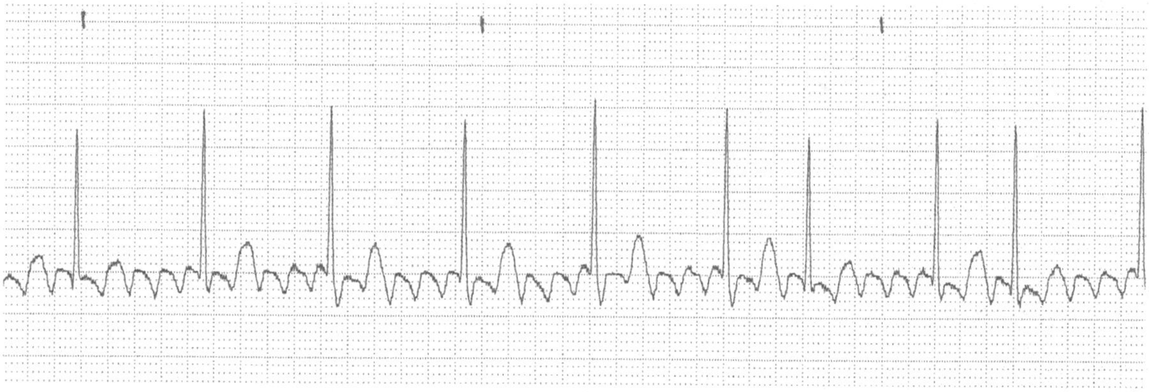

Strip 13.61. Rhythm: _____ Rate: _____ P wave: _____

PR interval: _____ QRS complex: _____

Rhythm interpretation: _____

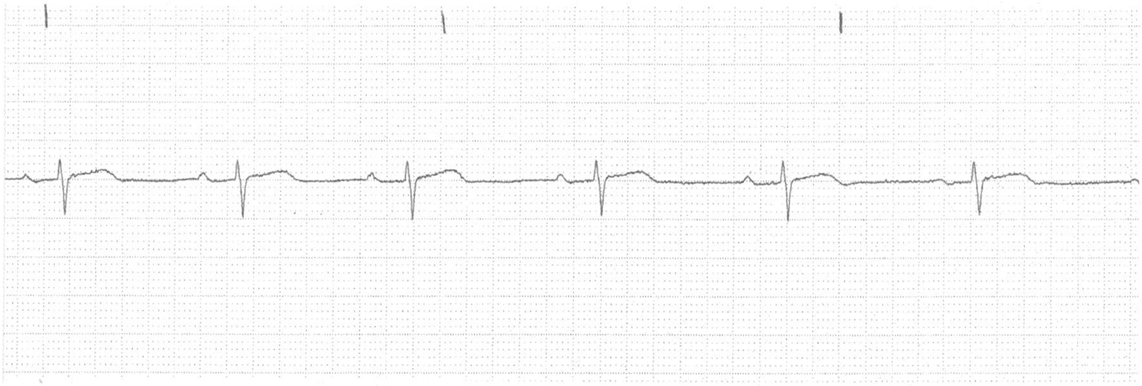

Strip 13.62. Rhythm: _____ Rate: _____ P wave: _____

PR interval: _____ QRS complex: _____

Rhythm interpretation: _____

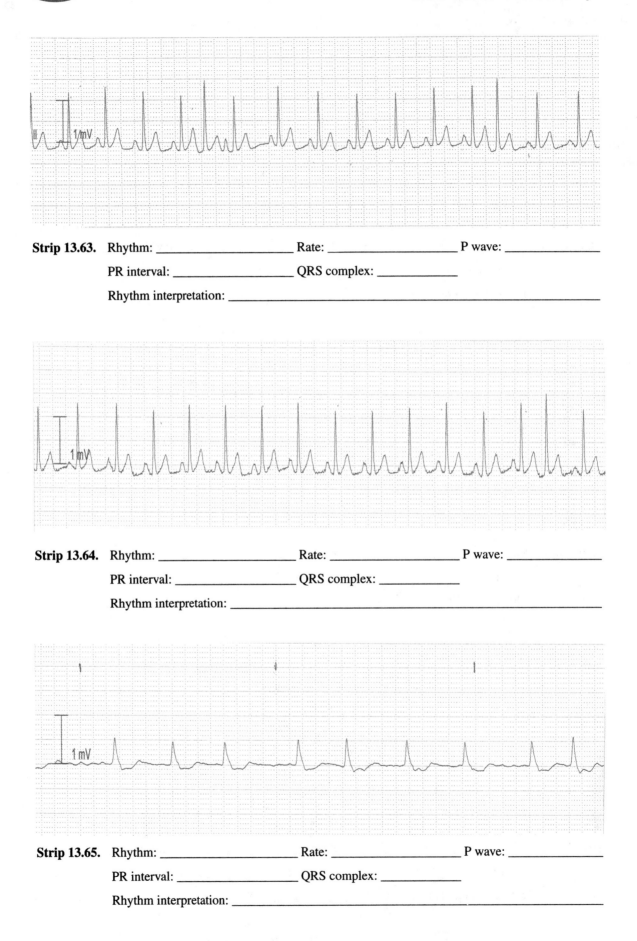

Strip 13.63. Rhythm: _____ Rate: _____ P wave: _____

PR interval: _____ QRS complex: _____

Rhythm interpretation: _____

Strip 13.64. Rhythm: _____ Rate: _____ P wave: _____

PR interval: _____ QRS complex: _____

Rhythm interpretation: _____

Strip 13.65. Rhythm: _____ Rate: _____ P wave: _____

PR interval: _____ QRS complex: _____

Rhythm interpretation: _____

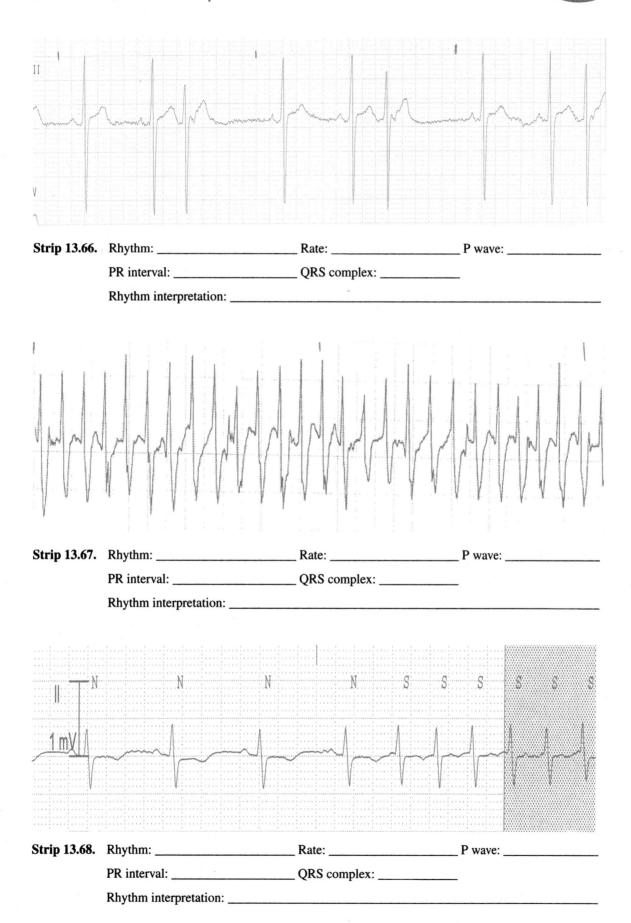

Strip 13.66. Rhythm: _____ Rate: _____ P wave: _____

PR interval: _____ QRS complex: _____

Rhythm interpretation: _____

Strip 13.67. Rhythm: _____ Rate: _____ P wave: _____

PR interval: _____ QRS complex: _____

Rhythm interpretation: _____

Strip 13.68. Rhythm: _____ Rate: _____ P wave: _____

PR interval: _____ QRS complex: _____

Rhythm interpretation: _____

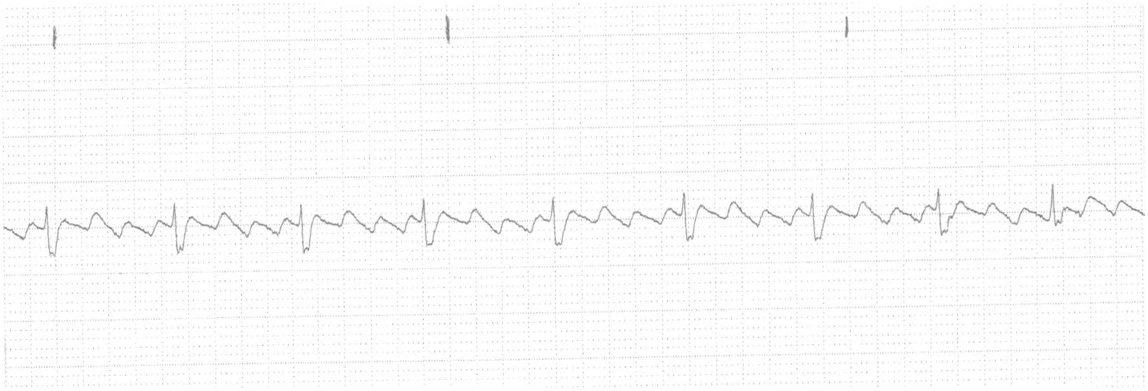

Strip 13.69. Rhythm: _____ Rate: _____ P wave: _____

PR interval: _____ QRS complex: _____

Rhythm interpretation: _____

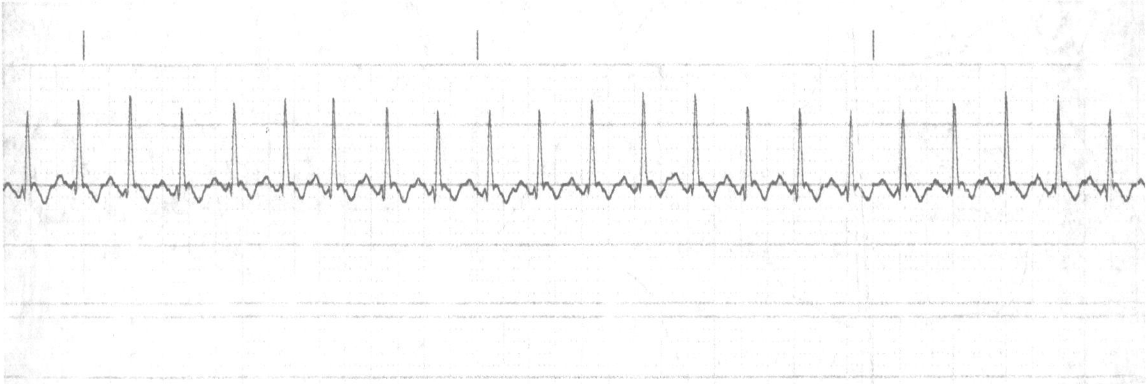

Strip 13.70. Rhythm: _____ Rate: _____ P wave: _____

PR interval: _____ QRS complex: _____

Rhythm interpretation: _____

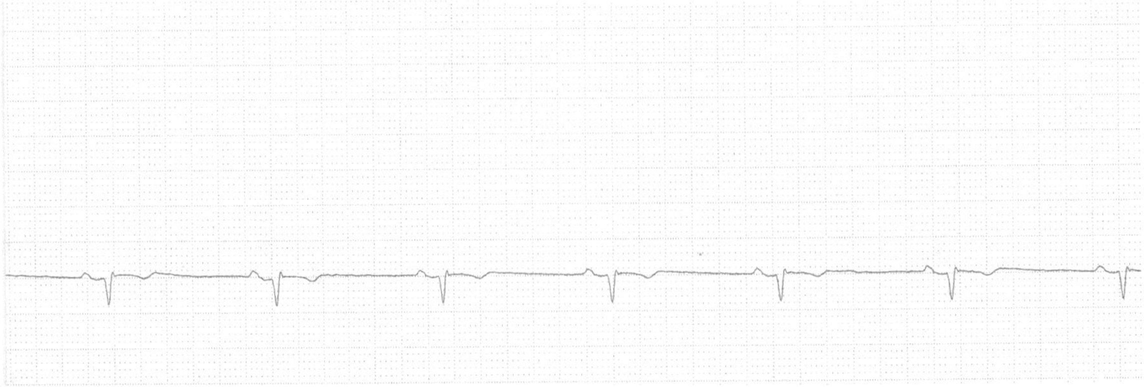

Strip 13.71. Rhythm: _____ Rate: _____ P wave: _____

PR interval: _____ QRS complex: _____

Rhythm interpretation: _____

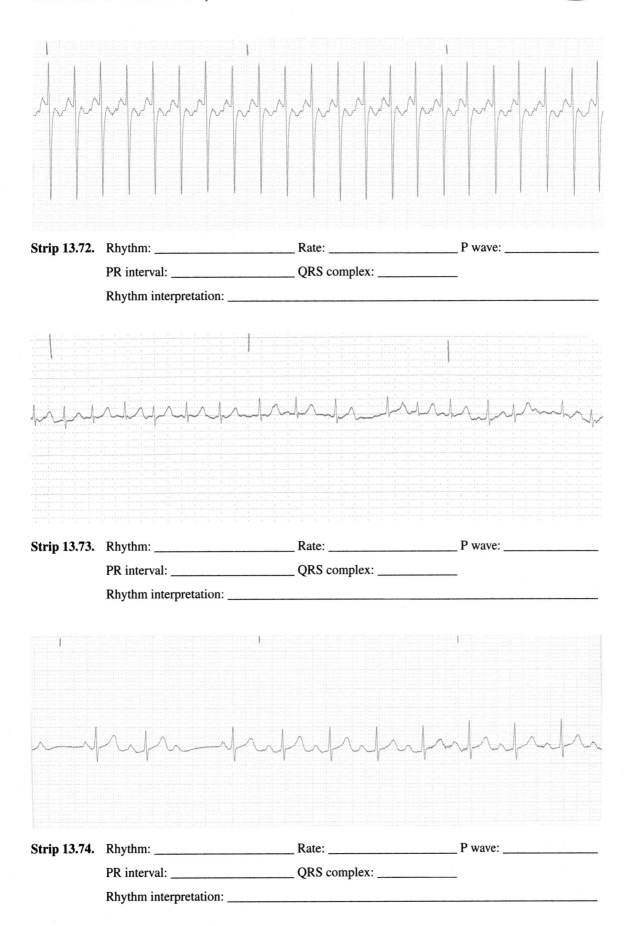

Strip 13.72. Rhythm: _____ Rate: _____ P wave: _____

PR interval: _____ QRS complex: _____

Rhythm interpretation: _____

Strip 13.73. Rhythm: _____ Rate: _____ P wave: _____

PR interval: _____ QRS complex: _____

Rhythm interpretation: _____

Strip 13.74. Rhythm: _____ Rate: _____ P wave: _____

PR interval: _____ QRS complex: _____

Rhythm interpretation: _____

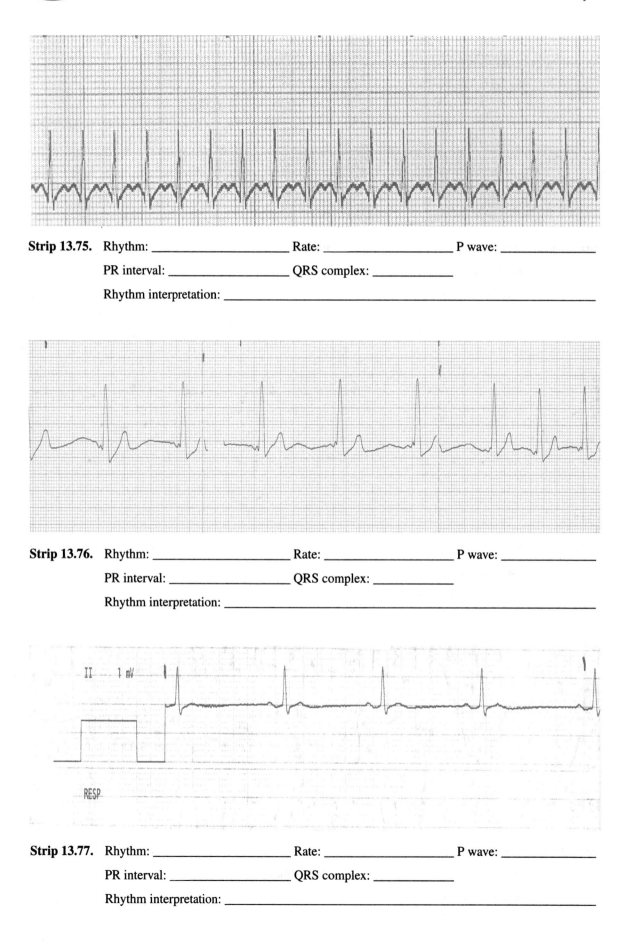

Strip 13.75. Rhythm: _____ Rate: _____ P wave: _____

PR interval: _____ QRS complex: _____

Rhythm interpretation: _____

Strip 13.76. Rhythm: _____ Rate: _____ P wave: _____

PR interval: _____ QRS complex: _____

Rhythm interpretation: _____

Strip 13.77. Rhythm: _____ Rate: _____ P wave: _____

PR interval: _____ QRS complex: _____

Rhythm interpretation: _____

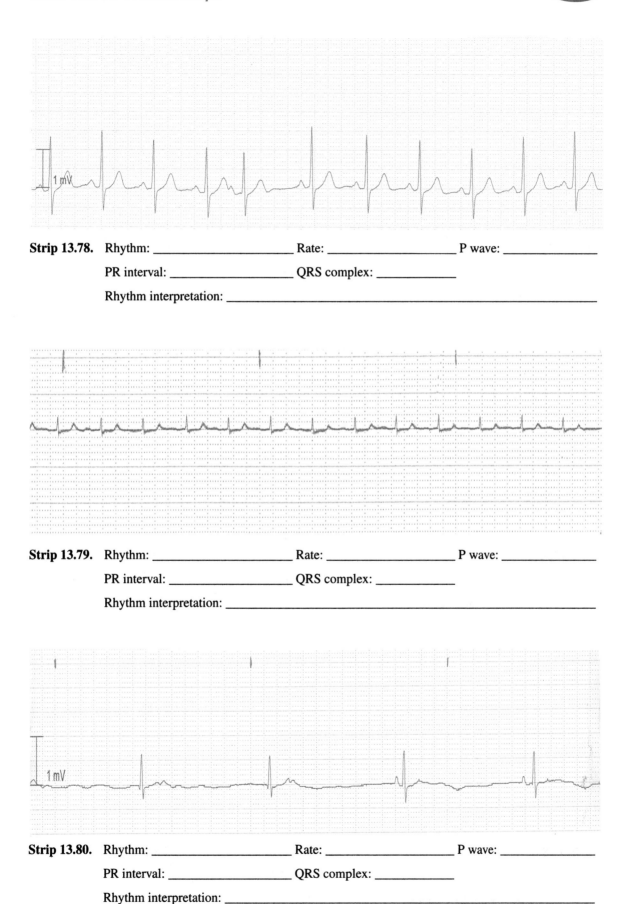

Strip 13.78. Rhythm: _____ Rate: _____ P wave: _____

PR interval: _____ QRS complex: _____

Rhythm interpretation: _____

Strip 13.79. Rhythm: _____ Rate: _____ P wave: _____

PR interval: _____ QRS complex: _____

Rhythm interpretation: _____

Strip 13.80. Rhythm: _____ Rate: _____ P wave: _____

PR interval: _____ QRS complex: _____

Rhythm interpretation: _____

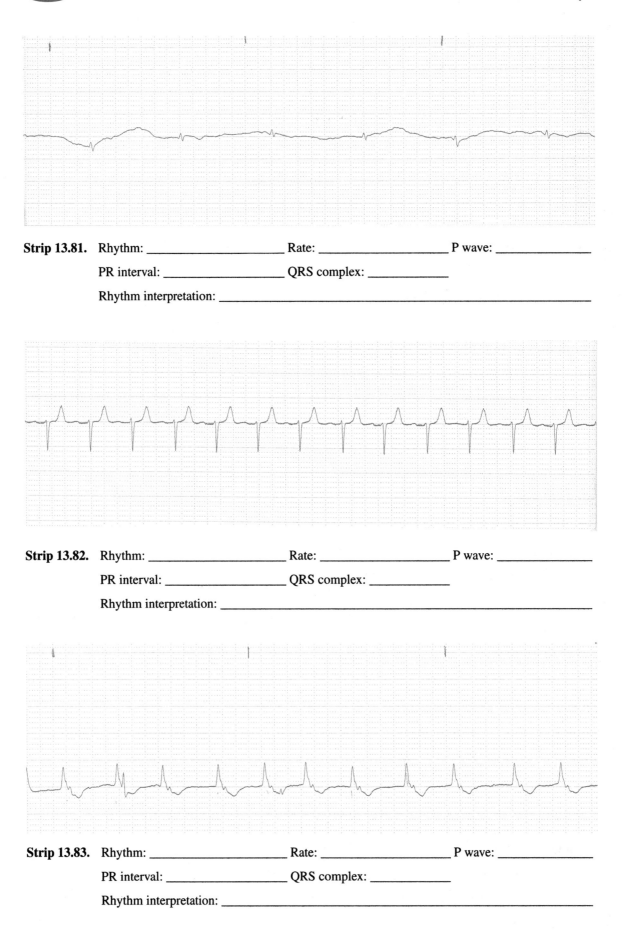

Strip 13.81. Rhythm: _____ Rate: _____ P wave: _____

PR interval: _____ QRS complex: _____

Rhythm interpretation: _____

Strip 13.82. Rhythm: _____ Rate: _____ P wave: _____

PR interval: _____ QRS complex: _____

Rhythm interpretation: _____

Strip 13.83. Rhythm: _____ Rate: _____ P wave: _____

PR interval: _____ QRS complex: _____

Rhythm interpretation: _____

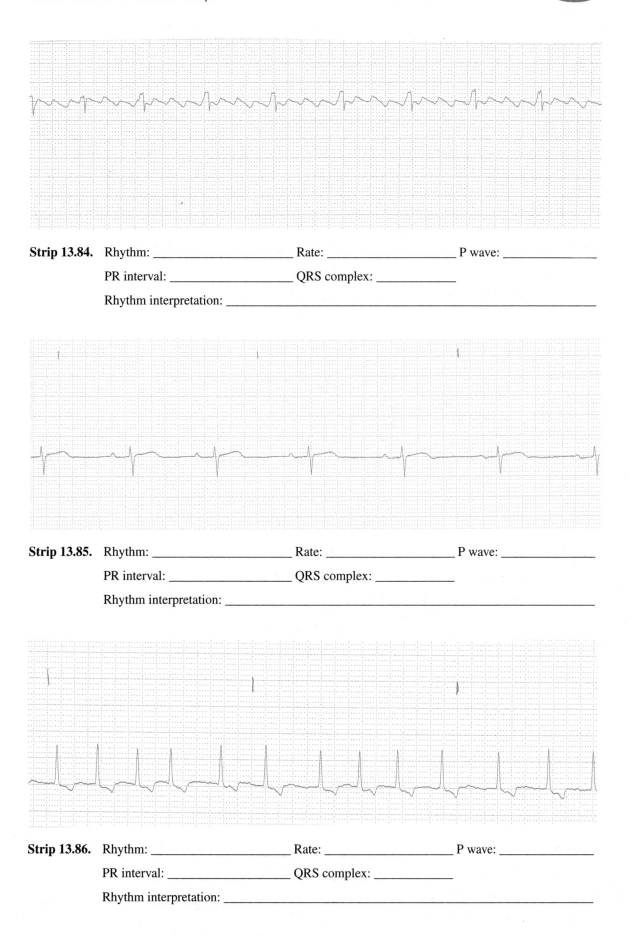

Strip 13.84. Rhythm: _____ Rate: _____ P wave: _____

PR interval: _____ QRS complex: _____

Rhythm interpretation: _____

Strip 13.85. Rhythm: _____ Rate: _____ P wave: _____

PR interval: _____ QRS complex: _____

Rhythm interpretation: _____

Strip 13.86. Rhythm: _____ Rate: _____ P wave: _____

PR interval: _____ QRS complex: _____

Rhythm interpretation: _____

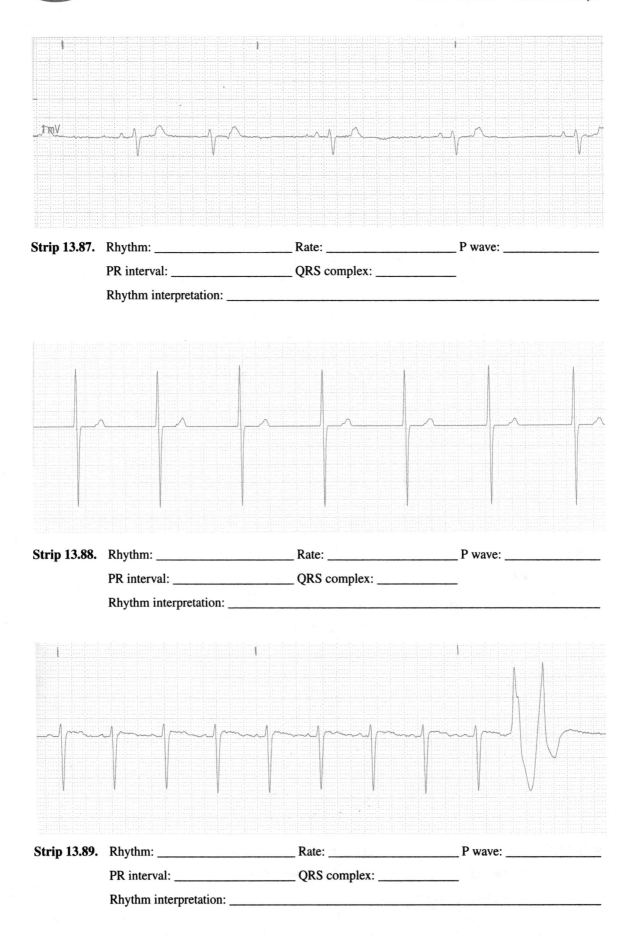

Strip 13.87. Rhythm: _____ Rate: _____ P wave: _____

PR interval: _____ QRS complex: _____

Rhythm interpretation: _____

Strip 13.88. Rhythm: _____ Rate: _____ P wave: _____

PR interval: _____ QRS complex: _____

Rhythm interpretation: _____

Strip 13.89. Rhythm: _____ Rate: _____ P wave: _____

PR interval: _____ QRS complex: _____

Rhythm interpretation: _____

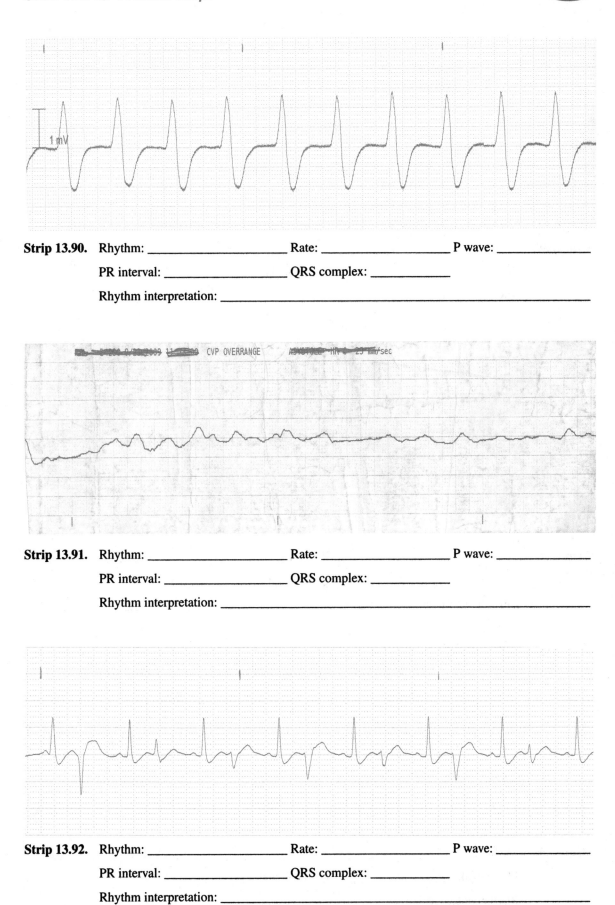

Strip 13.90. Rhythm: _____ Rate: _____ P wave: _____

PR interval: _____ QRS complex: _____

Rhythm interpretation: _____

Strip 13.91. Rhythm: _____ Rate: _____ P wave: _____

PR interval: _____ QRS complex: _____

Rhythm interpretation: _____

Strip 13.92. Rhythm: _____ Rate: _____ P wave: _____

PR interval: _____ QRS complex: _____

Rhythm interpretation: _____

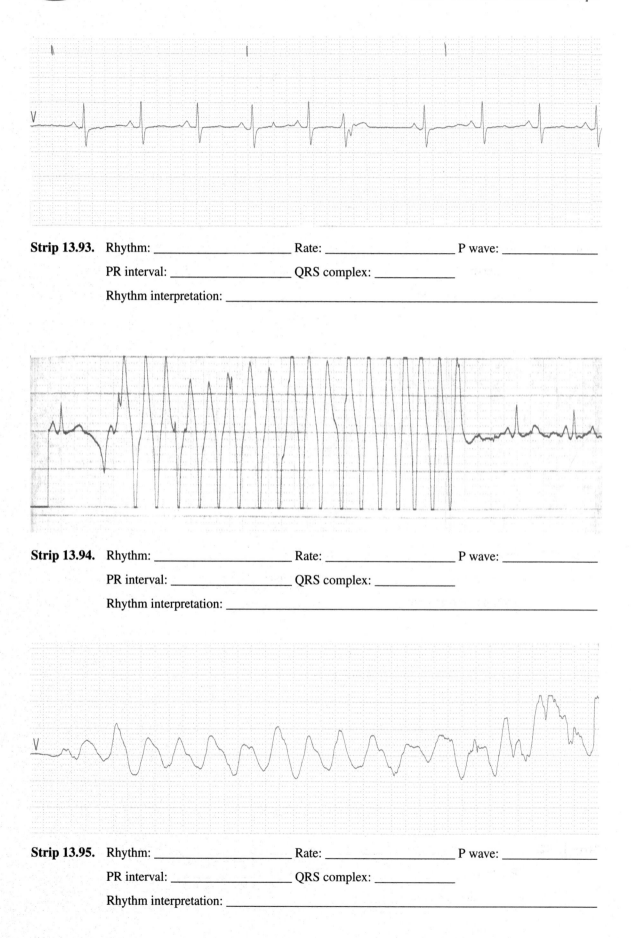

Strip 13.93. Rhythm: _____ Rate: _____ P wave: _____

PR interval: _____ QRS complex: _____

Rhythm interpretation: _____

Strip 13.94. Rhythm: _____ Rate: _____ P wave: _____

PR interval: _____ QRS complex: _____

Rhythm interpretation: _____

Strip 13.95. Rhythm: _____ Rate: _____ P wave: _____

PR interval: _____ QRS complex: _____

Rhythm interpretation: _____

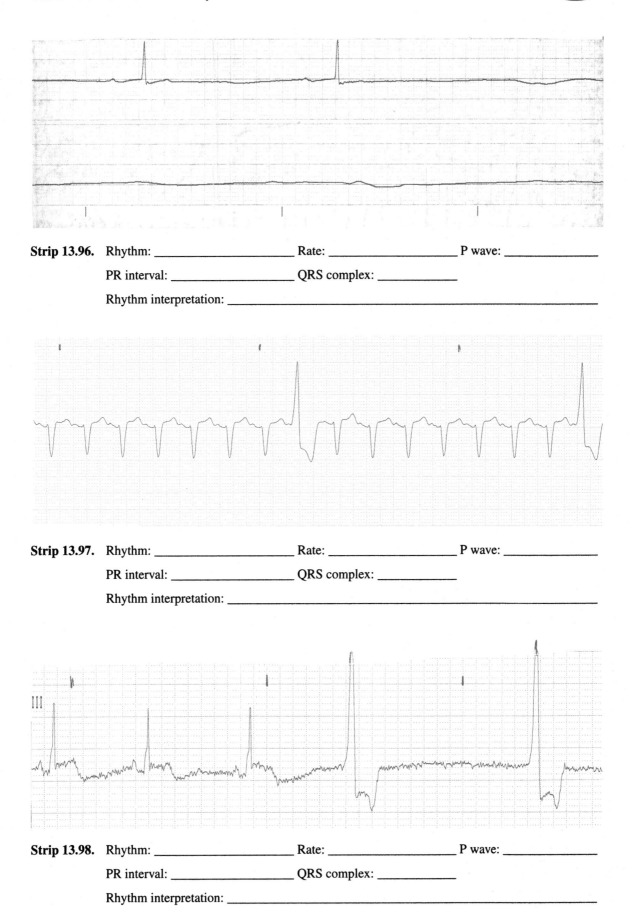

Strip 13.96. Rhythm: _____ Rate: _____ P wave: _____

PR interval: _____ QRS complex: _____

Rhythm interpretation: _____

Strip 13.97. Rhythm: _____ Rate: _____ P wave: _____

PR interval: _____ QRS complex: _____

Rhythm interpretation: _____

Strip 13.98. Rhythm: _____ Rate: _____ P wave: _____

PR interval: _____ QRS complex: _____

Rhythm interpretation: _____

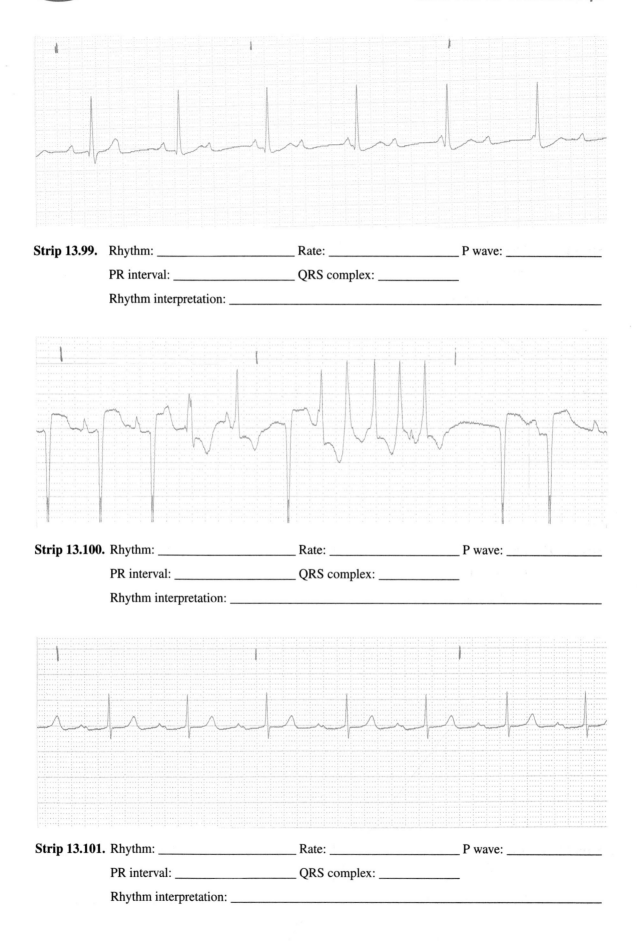

Strip 13.99. Rhythm: _____ Rate: _____ P wave: _____

PR interval: _____ QRS complex: _____

Rhythm interpretation: _____

Strip 13.100. Rhythm: _____ Rate: _____ P wave: _____

PR interval: _____ QRS complex: _____

Rhythm interpretation: _____

Strip 13.101. Rhythm: _____ Rate: _____ P wave: _____

PR interval: _____ QRS complex: _____

Rhythm interpretation: _____

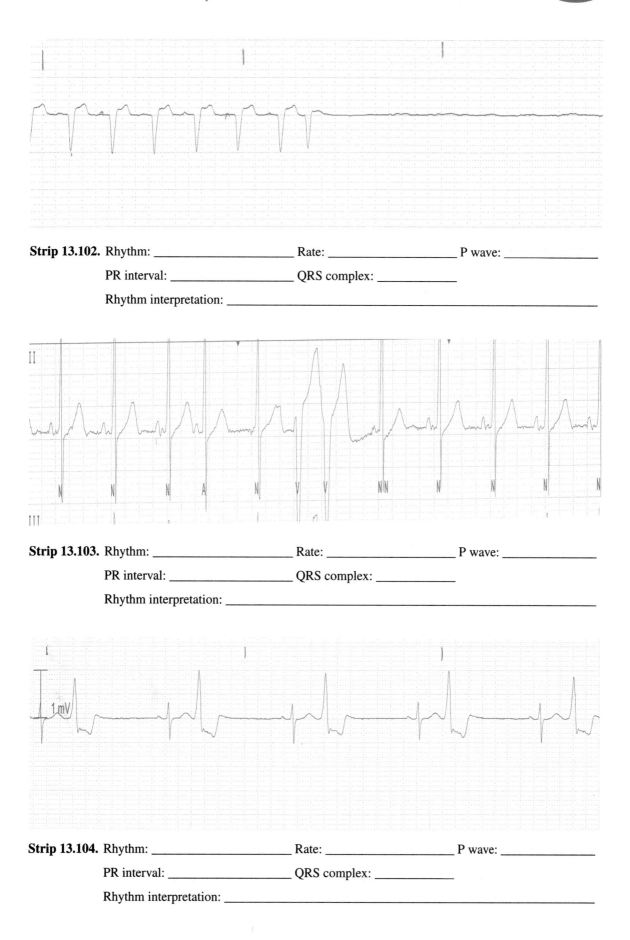

Strip 13.102. Rhythm: _____ Rate: _____ P wave: _____

PR interval: _____ QRS complex: _____

Rhythm interpretation: _____

Strip 13.103. Rhythm: _____ Rate: _____ P wave: _____

PR interval: _____ QRS complex: _____

Rhythm interpretation: _____

Strip 13.104. Rhythm: _____ Rate: _____ P wave: _____

PR interval: _____ QRS complex: _____

Rhythm interpretation: _____

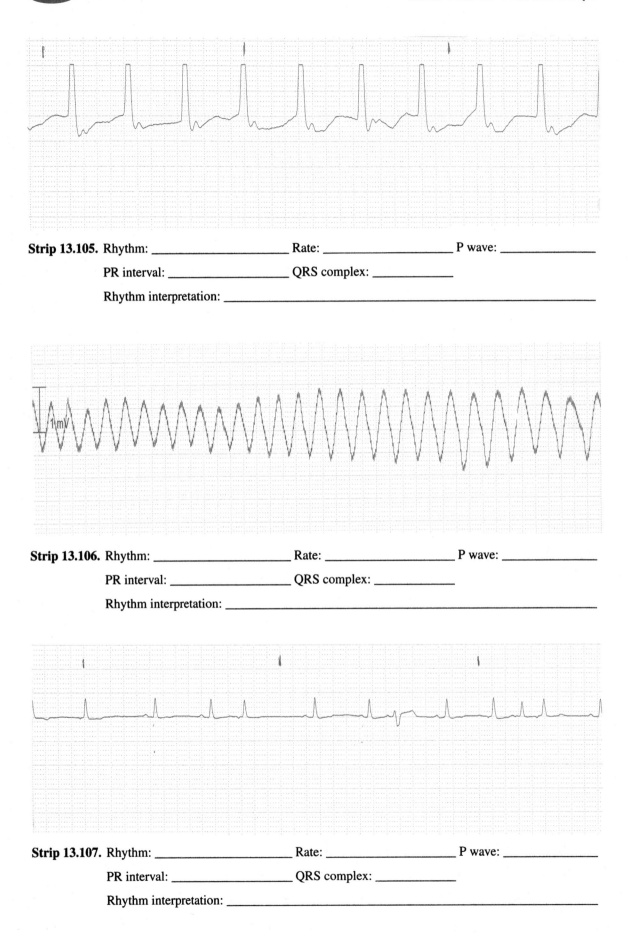

Strip 13.105. Rhythm: _____ Rate: _____ P wave: _____

PR interval: _____ QRS complex: _____

Rhythm interpretation: _____

Strip 13.106. Rhythm: _____ Rate: _____ P wave: _____

PR interval: _____ QRS complex: _____

Rhythm interpretation: _____

Strip 13.107. Rhythm: _____ Rate: _____ P wave: _____

PR interval: _____ QRS complex: _____

Rhythm interpretation: _____

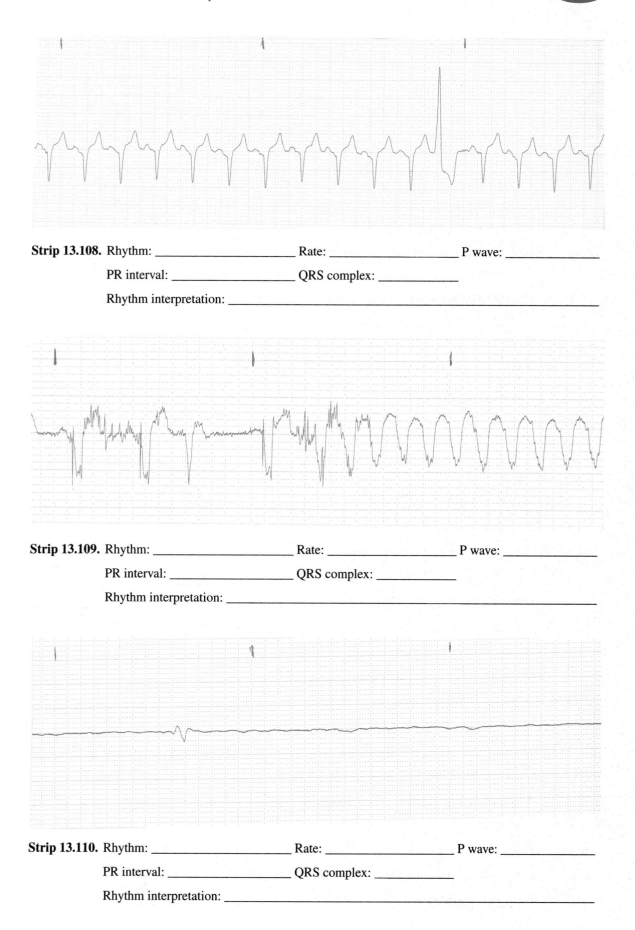

Strip 13.108. Rhythm: _____ Rate: _____ P wave: _____

PR interval: _____ QRS complex: _____

Rhythm interpretation: _____

Strip 13.109. Rhythm: _____ Rate: _____ P wave: _____

PR interval: _____ QRS complex: _____

Rhythm interpretation: _____

Strip 13.110. Rhythm: _____ Rate: _____ P wave: _____

PR interval: _____ QRS complex: _____

Rhythm interpretation: _____

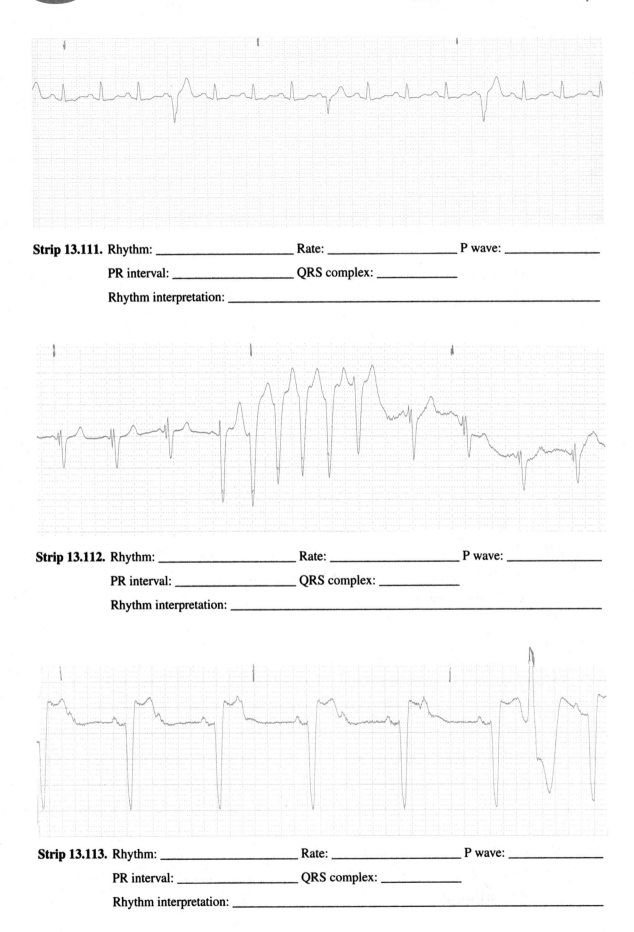

Strip 13.111. Rhythm: _____ Rate: _____ P wave: _____

PR interval: _____ QRS complex: _____

Rhythm interpretation: _____

Strip 13.112. Rhythm: _____ Rate: _____ P wave: _____

PR interval: _____ QRS complex: _____

Rhythm interpretation: _____

Strip 13.113. Rhythm: _____ Rate: _____ P wave: _____

PR interval: _____ QRS complex: _____

Rhythm interpretation: _____

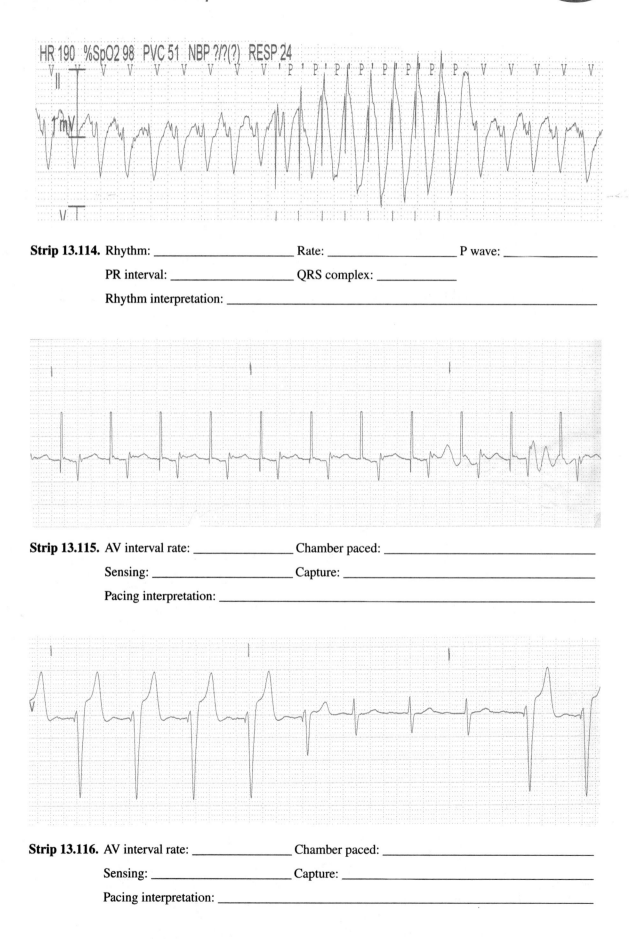

Strip 13.114. Rhythm: _____ Rate: _____ P wave: _____

PR interval: _____ QRS complex: _____

Rhythm interpretation: _____

Strip 13.115. AV interval rate: _____ Chamber paced: _____

Sensing: _____ Capture: _____

Pacing interpretation: _____

Strip 13.116. AV interval rate: _____ Chamber paced: _____

Sensing: _____ Capture: _____

Pacing interpretation: _____

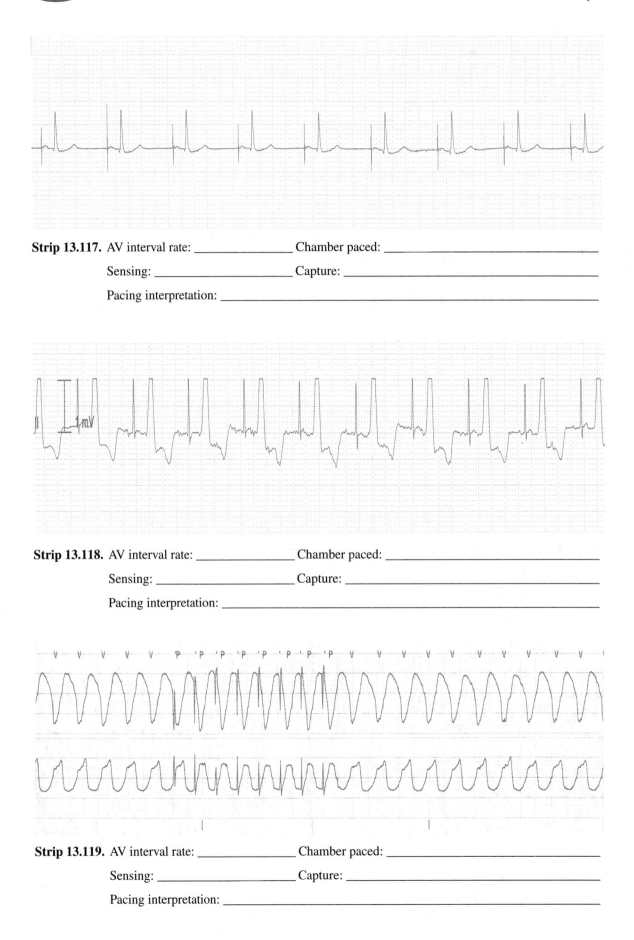

Strip 13.117. AV interval rate: _____ Chamber paced: _____

Sensing: _____ Capture: _____

Pacing interpretation: _____

Strip 13.118. AV interval rate: _____ Chamber paced: _____

Sensing: _____ Capture: _____

Pacing interpretation: _____

Strip 13.119. AV interval rate: _____ Chamber paced: _____

Sensing: _____ Capture: _____

Pacing interpretation: _____

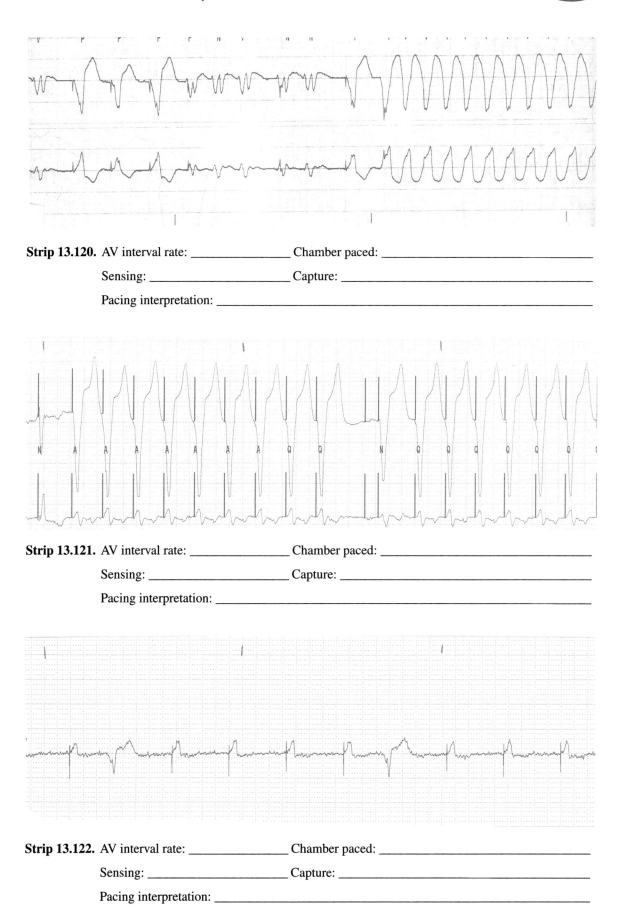

Strip 13.120. AV interval rate: _____ Chamber paced: _____

Sensing: _____ Capture: _____

Pacing interpretation: _____

Strip 13.121. AV interval rate: _____ Chamber paced: _____

Sensing: _____ Capture: _____

Pacing interpretation: _____

Strip 13.122. AV interval rate: _____ Chamber paced: _____

Sensing: _____ Capture: _____

Pacing interpretation: _____

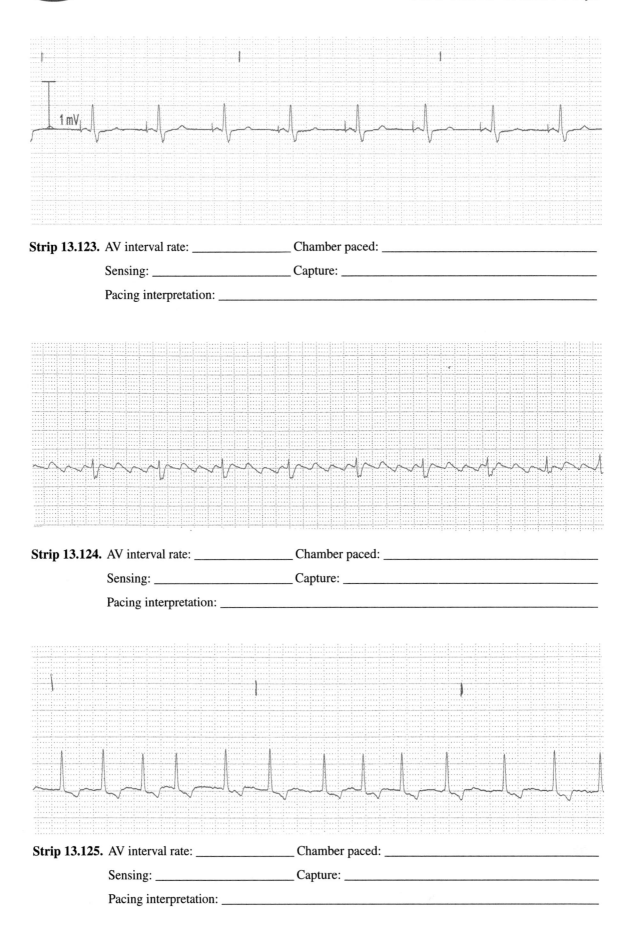

Strip 13.123. AV interval rate: _____ Chamber paced: _____

Sensing: _____ Capture: _____

Pacing interpretation: _____

Strip 13.124. AV interval rate: _____ Chamber paced: _____

Sensing: _____ Capture: _____

Pacing interpretation: _____

Strip 13.125. AV interval rate: _____ Chamber paced: _____

Sensing: _____ Capture: _____

Pacing interpretation: _____

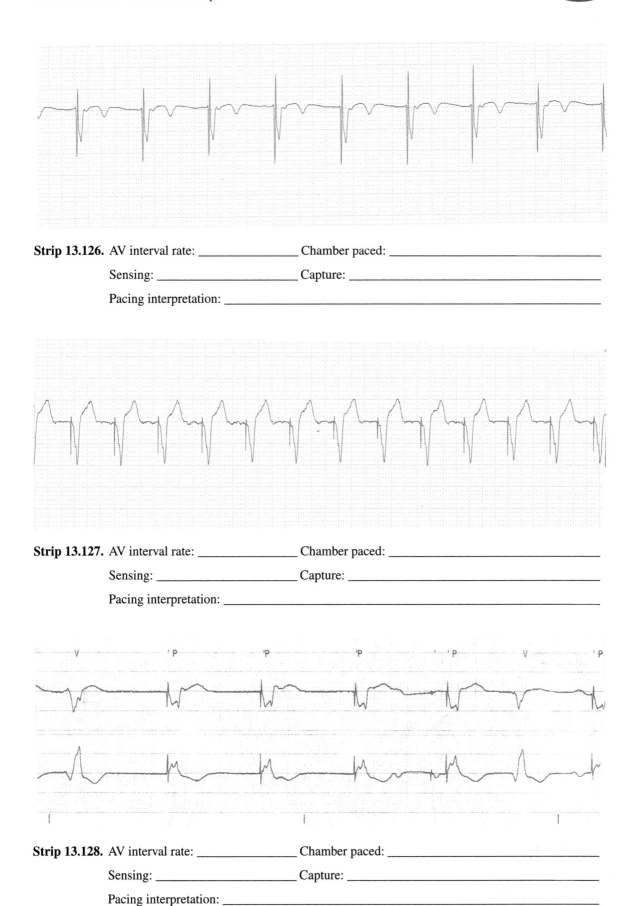

Strip 13.126. AV interval rate: _____ Chamber paced: _____

Sensing: _____ Capture: _____

Pacing interpretation: _____

Strip 13.127. AV interval rate: _____ Chamber paced: _____

Sensing: _____ Capture: _____

Pacing interpretation: _____

Strip 13.128. AV interval rate: _____ Chamber paced: _____

Sensing: _____ Capture: _____

Pacing interpretation: _____

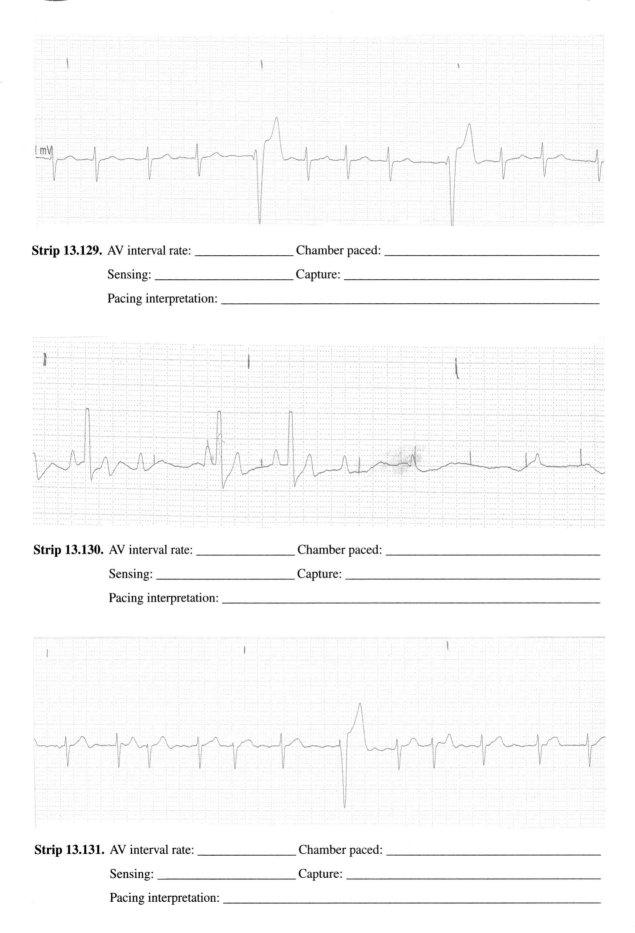

Strip 13.129. AV interval rate: _____ Chamber paced: _____

Sensing: _____ Capture: _____

Pacing interpretation: _____

Strip 13.130. AV interval rate: _____ Chamber paced: _____

Sensing: _____ Capture: _____

Pacing interpretation: _____

Strip 13.131. AV interval rate: _____ Chamber paced: _____

Sensing: _____ Capture: _____

Pacing interpretation: _____

Answer Key

Strip 13.1
Rhythm: Regular
Rate: 54
P wave: Sinus/notched
PR interval: 0.36
QRS complex: 0.08
Rhythm interpretation: Sinus bradycardia with
   1st degree

Strip 13.2
Rhythm: Irregular
Rate: 60
P wave: Sinus
PR interval: 0.16
QRS complex: 0.08
Rhythm interpretation: Sinus arrhythmia

Strip 13.3
Rhythm: Regular
Rate: 80
P wave: Sinus
PR interval: 0.20
QRS complex: 0.06
Rhythm interpretation: Normal sinus rhythm

Strip 13.4
Rhythm: Regular
Rate: 68
P wave: Sinus
PR interval: 0.16
QRS complex: 0.08
Rhythm interpretation: Normal sinus rhythm

Strip 13.5
Rhythm: Regular
Rate: 75
P wave: Sinus
PR interval: 0.20
QRS complex: 0.08
Rhythm interpretation: Normal sinus rhythm

Strip 13.6
Rhythm: Regular
Rate: 88
P wave: Sinus
PR interval: 0.20
QRS complex: 0.08
Rhythm interpretation: Normal sinus rhythm

Strip 13.7
Rhythm: Regular
Rate: 115
P wave: Sinus
PR interval: 0.16
QRS complex: 0.06
Rhythm interpretation: Sinus tachycardia

Strip 13.8
Rhythm: Irregular
Rate: 115
P wave: Sinus
PR interval: 0.12
QRS complex: 0.08
Rhythm interpretation: Sinus tachycardia with
   1 premature atrial contraction

Strip 13.9
Rhythm: Regular
Rate: 88
P wave: Sinus
PR interval: 0.16
QRS complex: 0.08
Rhythm interpretation: Normal sinus rhythm

Strip 13.10
Rhythm: Regular
Rate: 115
P wave: Sinus
PR interval: 0.20
QRS complex: 0.04
Rhythm interpretation: Sinus tachycardia

Strip 13.11
Rhythm: Regular
Rate: 63
P wave: Sinus
PR interval: 0.12
QRS complex: 0.06
Rhythm interpretation: Normal sinus rhythm

Strip 13.12
Rhythm: Irregular
Rate: 125
P wave: Sinus
PR interval: 0.12
QRS complex: 0.08
Rhythm interpretation: Sinus tachycardia with
   1 premature atrial contraction

Strip 13.13
Rhythm: Regular
Rate: 68
P wave: Sinus
PR interval: 0.16
QRS complex: 0.04
Rhythm interpretation: Normal sinus rhythm

Strip 13.14
Rhythm: Regular
Rate: 72
P wave: Sinus
PR interval: 0.15
QRS complex: 0.12
Rhythm interpretation: Normal sinus rhythm

Strip 13.15
Rhythm: Regular
Rate: 150
P wave: Sinus
PR interval: 0.16
QRS complex: 0.04
Rhythm interpretation: Sinus tachycardia

Strip 13.16
Rhythm: Regular
Rate: 88
P wave: Sinus
PR interval: 0.12
QRS complex: 0.06
Rhythm interpretation: Normal sinus rhythm

Strip 13.17
Rhythm: Regular
Rate: 125
P wave: Sinus
PR interval: 0.16
QRS complex: 0.08
Rhythm interpretation: Sinus tachycardia

Strip 13.18
Rhythm: Regular
Rate: 47
P wave: Sinus/notched
PR interval: 0.20
QRS complex: 0.06
Rhythm interpretation: Sinus bradycardia

Strip 13.19
Rhythm: Irregular
Rate: 111
P wave: Sinus
PR interval: 0.20
QRS complex: 0.08
Rhythm interpretation: Sinus tachycardia with premature atrial contractions

Strip 13.20
Rhythm: Regular
Rate: 115
P wave: Sinus
PR interval: 0.16
QRS complex: 0.08
Rhythm interpretation: Sinus tachycardia

Strip 13.21
Rhythm: Irregular
Rate: 60
P wave: Sinus
PR interval: 0.14
QRS complex: 0.08
Rhythm interpretation: Sinus arrhythmia

Strip 13.22
Rhythm: Regular
Rate: 115
P wave: Sinus
PR interval: 0.12
QRS complex: 0.12
Rhythm interpretation: Sinus tachycardia

Strip 13.23
Rhythm: Regular
Rate: 60
P wave: Sinus
PR interval: 0.12
QRS complex: 0.04
Rhythm interpretation: Normal sinus rhythm

Strip 13.24
Rhythm: Regular
Rate: 88
P wave: Sinus
PR interval: 0.12
QRS complex: 0.04
Rhythm interpretation: Normal sinus rhythm

Strip 13.25
Rhythm: Regular
Rate: 52
P wave: Sinus
PR interval: 0.16
QRS complex: 0.08
Rhythm interpretation: Sinus bradycardia

Strip 13.26
Rhythm: Irregular
Rate: 40
P wave: Sinus
PR interval: 0.20
QRS complex: 0.10
Rhythm interpretation: Sinus bradycardia arrhythmia

Strip 13.27
Rhythm: Regular
Rate: 56
P wave: 2 P's for every QRS, sinus
PR interval: 0.12
QRS complex: 0.06
Rhythm interpretation: 2nd degree type II with a
    2:1 conduction

Strip 13.28
Rhythm: Regular
Rate: 36
P wave: 3 P's for every QRS, sinus
PR interval: 0.28
QRS complex: 0.08
Rhythm interpretation: 2nd degree type II with a
    3:1 conduction

Strip 13.29
Rhythm: Irregular
Rate: 60
P wave: Sinus
PR interval: 0.32-0.44
QRS complex: 0.08
Rhythm interpretation: 2nd degree type I

Strip 13.30
Rhythm: Irregular
Rate: 50
P wave: Sinus 2:1 QRS
PR interval: 0.22
QRS complex: 0.10
Rhythm interpretation: 2nd degree type II

Strip 13.31
Rhythm: Regular
Rate: 84
P wave: Sinus
PR interval: 0.16
QRS complex: 0.06
Rhythm interpretation: Normal sinus rhythm

Strip 13.32
Rhythm: Regular
Rate: 79
P wave: P wave after the QRS
PR interval: N/A
QRS complex: 0.10
Rhythm interpretation: Accelerated junctional

Strip 13.33
Rhythm: Regular
Rate: 95
P wave: Sinus, extra P wave after the 10th complex
PR interval: 0.28
QRS complex: 0.04
Rhythm interpretation: Normal sinus rhythm with a
    1st degree and non conducted premature atrial con-
    traction after the 10th complex

Strip 13.34
Rhythm: Irregular
Rate: 40
P wave: Sinus, no relation to the QRS
PR interval: N/A
QRS complex: 0.08
Rhythm interpretation: Complete heart block

Strip 13.35
Rhythm: Irregular
Rate: 80
P wave: Sinus
PR interval: 0.24
QRS complex: 0.06
Rhythm interpretation: Normal sinus rhythm with
    1st degree frequent premature atrial contraction 2,
    4, 7, 9th complex

Strip 13.36
Rhythm: Irregular
Rate: 70
P wave: Flutter
PR interval: N/A
QRS complex: 0.04
Rhythm interpretation: Atrial flutter 5:1 conduction

Strip 13.37
Rhythm: Regular
Rate: 56
P wave: Sinus 2:1 P:QRS
PR interval: 0.12
QRS complex: 0.06
Rhythm interpretation: 2nd degree type II 2:1
    conduction

Strip 13.38
Rhythm: Regular
Rate: 30
P wave: Sinus but no relation to the QRS
PR interval: N/A
QRS complex: 0.12
Rhythm interpretation: Complete heart block

Strip 13.39
Rhythm: Regular
Rate: 68
P wave: Sinus
PR interval: 0.36
QRS complex: 0.06
Rhythm interpretation: Normal sinus rhythm with a
1st degree block

Strip 13.40
Rhythm: Regular
Rate: 150
P wave: Hidden by the T wave
PR interval: N/A
QRS complex: 0.06
Rhythm interpretation: Supraventricular tachycardia

Strip 13.41
Rhythm: Regular
Rate: 40
P wave: Sinus
PR interval: 0.24
QRS complex: 0.08
Rhythm interpretation: Sinus bradycardia with a
1st degree

Strip 13.42
Rhythm: Regular
Rate: 34
P wave: Sinus, with 3 P's to every QRS
PR interval: 0.32
QRS complex: 0.06
Rhythm interpretation: Second degree type II, 3:1
conduction

Strip 13.43
Rhythm: Irregular
Rate: 30
P wave: Sinus, non relation to the QRS
PR interval: N/A
QRS complex: 0.08
Rhythm interpretation: Complete heart block convert-
ing to a ventricular standstill

Strip 13.44
Rhythm: Irregular
Rate: 100
P wave: Fibrillatory
PR interval: N/A
QRS complex: 0.10
Rhythm interpretation: Controlled atrial fibrillation

Strip 13.45
Rhythm: Regular
Rate: 80
P wave: Sinus
PR interval: 0.28
QRS complex: 0.06
Rhythm interpretation: Normal sinus rhythm with a
1st degree block

Strip 13.46
Rhythm: Regular
Rate: 47-50
P wave: Varies in size and shape
PR interval: 0.24-0.26
QRS complex: 0.08
Rhythm interpretation: Wandering atrial pacemaker

Strip 13.47
Rhythm: Regular
Rate: 84
P wave: Sinus
PR interval: 0.20
QRS complex: 0.06
Rhythm interpretation: Normal sinus rhythm

Strip 13.48
Rhythm: Regular
Rate: 68
P wave: Indeterminable
PR interval: N/A
QRS complex: 0.06
Rhythm interpretation: Baseline distorted by artifact,
such as the patient is shaving with an electric shaver

Strip 13.49
Rhythm: Regular
Rate: 56
P wave: 2 P's for every QRS
PR interval: 0.16
QRS complex: 0.06
Rhythm interpretation: Second degree type II 2:1
conduction

Strip 13.50
Rhythm: Regular
Rate: 102
P wave: Not present (U wave is visible)
PR interval: N/A
QRS complex: 0.04
Rhythm interpretation: Junctional tachycardia

Strip 13.51
Rhythm: Irregular
Rate: 100
P wave: Fibrillatory
PR interval: N/A
QRS complex: 0.08
Rhythm interpretation: Controlled atrial fibrillation

Strip 13.52
Rhythm: Regular
Rate: 80
P wave: Sinus
PR interval: 0.16
QRS complex: 0.08
Rhythm interpretation: Normal sinus rhythm with 1 premature atrial contraction after 3rd complex

Strip 13.53
Rhythm: Regular
Rate: 94
P wave: Sinus
PR interval: 0.24
QRS complex: 0.08
Rhythm interpretation: Normal sinus rhythm with 1 nonconducted premature atrial contraction after the 4th complex

Strip 13.54
Rhythm: Regular
Rate: 65
P wave: Flutter
PR interval: N/A
QRS complex: 0.06
Rhythm interpretation: Atrial flutter 4:1 conduction

Strip 13.55
Rhythm: Irregular
Rate: 100
P wave: Fibrillatory
PR interval: N/A
QRS complex: 0.08
Rhythm interpretation: Controlled atrial fibrillation

Strip 13.56
Rhythm: Irregular
Rate: 130
P wave: Sinus
PR interval: 0.18
QRS complex: 0.04
Rhythm interpretation: A sinus beat then 1 premature atrial contraction, then sinus beat, premature ventricular contraction, burst of afibrillation, sinus beat, 1 premature atrial contraction ending with a sinus beat

Strip 13.57
Rhythm: Irregular
Rate: 110
P wave: Fibrillatory
PR interval: N/A
QRS complex: 0.08
Rhythm interpretation: Rapid or uncontrolled atrial fibrillation

Strip 13.58
Rhythm: Irregular
Rate: 60
P wave: Fibrillatory
PR interval: N/A
QRS complex: 0.04
Rhythm interpretation: Controlled atrial fibrillation

Strip 13.59
Rhythm: Irregular
Rate: 40
P wave: Fibrillatory
PR interval: N/A
QRS complex: 0.04
Rhythm interpretation: Controlled atrial fibrillation

Strip 13.60
Rhythm: Regular
Rate: 214
P wave: Hidden in the T waves
PR interval: Immeasurable
QRS complex: 0.06
Rhythm interpretation: Supraventricular tachycardia

Strip 13.61
Rhythm: Irregular
Rate: 70
P wave: Flutter
PR interval: Immeasurable
QRS complex: 0.08
Rhythm interpretation: Atrial flutter with varying conduction

Strip 13.62
Rhythm: Regular
Rate: 48
P wave: Varies in size and shape
PR interval: 0.32
QRS complex: 0.06
Rhythm interpretation: Wandering atrial pacemaker, bradycardia

Strip 13.63
Rhythm: Irregular
Rate: 113
P wave: Sinus
PR interval: 0.12
QRS complex: 0.08
Rhythm interpretation: Sinus tachycardia with premature atrial contraction after the 5th and 14th complex

Strip 13.64
Rhythm: Regular
Rate: 113
P wave: Sinus
PR interval: 0.16
QRS complex: 0.04
Rhythm interpretation: Sinus tachycardia with premature atrial contraction after the 14th complex

Strip 13.65
Rhythm: Regular
Rate: 70
P wave: Fibrillatory
PR interval: N/A
QRS complex: 0.12
Rhythm interpretation: Controlled atrial fibrillation

Strip 13.66
Rhythm: Irregular
Rate: 60
P wave: Sinus
PR interval: 0.20
QRS complex: 0.10
Rhythm interpretation: Normal sinus rhythm with frequent premature atrial contraction or atrial trigeminy

Strip 13.67
Rhythm: Regular
Rate: 250
P wave: Hidden in T waves
PR interval: Immeasurable
QRS complex: 0.08
Rhythm interpretation: Supraventricular tachycardia

Strip 13.68
Rhythm: Regular–Irregular
Rate: 56-120
P wave: Sinus–Fibrillatory
PR interval: 0.16
QRS complex: 0.10
Rhythm interpretation: Sinus bradycardia converting to an uncontrolled or rapid atrial fibrillation

Strip 13.69
Rhythm: Regular
Rate: 65
P wave: Flutter
PR interval: N/A
QRS complex: 0.12
Rhythm interpretation: Atrial flutter 4:1 conduction

Strip 13.70
Rhythm: Regular
Rate: 167
P wave: Hidden in T wave
PR interval: N/A
QRS complex: 0.06
Rhythm interpretation: Supraventricular tachycardia

Strip 13.71
Rhythm: Regular
Rate: 48
P wave: Sinus
PR interval: 0.20
QRS complex: 0.06
Rhythm interpretation: Sinus bradycardia

Strip 13.72
Rhythm: Regular
Rate: 150
P wave: Hidden in T wave
PR interval: N/A
QRS complex: 0.08
Rhythm interpretation: Supraventricular tachycardia

Strip 13.73
Rhythm: Irregular
Rate: 120
P wave: Fibrillatory
PR interval: N/A
QRS complex: 0.06
Rhythm interpretation: Rapid or uncontrolled atrial fibrillation

Strip 13.74
Rhythm: Irregular–Regular
Rate: 70
P wave: Sinus
PR interval: 0.20
QRS complex: 0.04
Rhythm interpretation: Normal sinus rhythm with nonconducted premature atrial contraction on 3rd beat

Strip 13.75
Rhythm: Irregular
Rate: 167
P wave: Hidden in T wave
PR interval: N/A
QRS complex: 0.06
Rhythm interpretation: Supraventricular tachycardia

Strip 13.76
Rhythm: Irregular
Rate: 59-94
P wave: In the beginning of the QRS
PR interval: N/A
QRS complex: 0.06
Rhythm interpretation: Junctional to accelerated
  junctional

Strip 13.77
Rhythm: Regular
Rate: 45
P wave: Sinus
PR interval: 0.20
QRS complex: 0.06
Rhythm interpretation: Sinus bradycardia

Strip 13.78
Rhythm: Regular
Rate: 75
P wave: Sinus
PR interval: 0.016
QRS complex: 0.08
Rhythm interpretation: Normal sinus rhythm with
  1 premature atrial contraction after the 4th complex

Strip 13.79
Rhythm: Regular
Rate: 88
P wave: Not present
PR interval: N/A
QRS complex: 0.04
Rhythm interpretation: Accelerated junctional

Strip 13.80
Rhythm: Regular
Rate: 32
P wave: Present after the QRS in the T wave after the 1st
  and 2nd complex, sinus on the 3rd and 4th complex
PR interval: Varies 0.10-0.12
QRS complex: 0.08
Rhythm interpretation: Junctional to sinus bradycardia

Strip 13.81
Rhythm: Regular
Rate: 44
P wave: Not present
PR interval: N/A
QRS complex: 0.06
Rhythm interpretation: Junctional

Strip 13.82
Rhythm: Regular
Rate: 100
P wave: Not present
PR interval: N/A
QRS complex: 0.04
Rhythm interpretation: Accelerated junctional

Strip 13.83
Rhythm: Irregular
Rate: 80
P wave: Present after the QRS
PR interval: N/A
QRS complex: 0.10
Rhythm interpretation: Accelerated junctional

Strip 13.84
Rhythm: Regular
Rate: 65
P wave: Flutter
PR interval: N/A
QRS complex: 0.12
Rhythm interpretation: Atrial flutter 4:1 conduction

Strip 13.85
Rhythm: Regular
Rate: 43
P wave: Varies in size and shape
PR interval: 0.28
QRS complex: 0.08
Rhythm interpretation: Wandering atrial pacemeaker

Strip 13.86
Rhythm: Irregular
Rate: 100
P wave: Fibrillatory
PR interval: N/A
QRS complex: 0.06
Rhythm interpretation: Atrial fibrillation

Strip 13.87
Rhythm: Irregular
Rate: 40
P wave: Sinus
PR interval: 0.20
QRS complex: 0.06
Rhythm interpretation: Sinus bradycardia with 1 pre-
  mature junctional complex after the 2nd complex

Strip 13.88
Rhythm: Regular
Rate: 47
P wave: After the QRS
PR interval: N/A
QRS complex: 0.08
Rhythm interpretation: Junctional

Strip 13.89
Rhythm: Regular
Rate: 80
P wave: Sinus
PR interval: 0.18
QRS complex: 0.08
Rhythm interpretation: Normal sinus rhythm with
  couplet premature ventricular contraction

Strip 13.90
Rhythm: Regular
Rate: 70
P wave: None
PR interval: N/A
QRS complex: 0.12
Rhythm interpretation: Accelerated idioventricular rhythm

Strip 13.91
Rhythm: Irregular
Rate: 0
P wave: 0
PR interval: 0
QRS complex: 0
Rhythm interpretation: Venticular fibrillation

Strip 13.92
Rhythm: Irregular
Rate: 60
P wave: Sinus
PR interval: 0.12
QRS complex: 0.08
Rhythm interpretation: Normal sinus rhythm with ventricular bigeminy

Strip 13.93
Rhythm: Regular–Irregular
Rate: 75
P wave: Sinus
PR interval: 0.20
QRS complex: 0.08
Rhythm interpretation: Normal sinus rhythm with 1 premature ventricular contraction

Strip 13.94
Rhythm: Irregular
Rate: 250
P wave: Occasional sinus
PR interval: On the sinus beats 0.16
QRS complex: 0.08
Rhythm interpretation: 1 sinus beat, 17 beats of ventricular tachycardia, followed by 2 sinus beats

Strip 13.95
Rhythm: Irregular
Rate: 0
P wave: 0
PR interval: 0
QRS complex: 0
Rhythm interpretation: Coarse ventricular fibrillation

Strip 13.96
Rhythm: Irregular
Rate: 21
P wave: Sinus
PR interval: 0.44
QRS complex: 0.06
Rhythm interpretation: Atrial escape rhythm

Strip 13.97
Rhythm: Regular
Rate: 125
P wave: Obscured by the T wave
PR interval: N/A
QRS complex: 0.08
Rhythm interpretation: Sinus tachycardia with 2 unifocal premature ventricular contraction

Strip 13.98
Rhythm: Regular–Irregular
Rate: 41-22
P wave: Sinus
PR interval: 0.24
QRS complex: 0.08
Rhythm interpretation: 3 atrial escape beats converting to an idioventricular rhythm

Strip 13.99
Rhythm: Regular
Rate: 43
P wave: Sinus, no relation to the QRS
PR interval: N/A
QRS complex: 0.08
Rhythm interpretation: Complete heart block

Strip 13.100
Rhythm: Irregular
Rate: First three beats 75
P wave: Varies
PR interval: 0.24
QRS complex: Varies
Rhythm interpretation: 2 sinus beats, 1 premature ventricular contraction, 1 atrial escape beat, 1 junctional escape beat, 5-beat run of ventricular tachycardia, junctional escape

Strip 13.101
Rhythm: Regular
Rate: 52
P wave: Sinus
PR interval: 0.44
QRS complex: 0.04
Rhythm interpretation: Sinus bradycardia with 1st degree

Strip 13.102
Rhythm: Irregular
Rate: Initially 100
P wave: Flattened
PR interval: 0.18
QRS complex: 0.08
Rhythm interpretation: Normal sinus rhythm to asystole

Strip 13.103
Rhythm: Irregular
Rate: 75
P wave: Sinus
PR interval: 0.16
QRS complex: 0.04
Rhythm interpretation: Normal sinus rhythm with premature atrial contraction and premature junctional complex, couplet

Strip 13.104
Rhythm: Irregular
Rate: 38
P wave: Sinus
PR interval: 0.20
QRS complex: 0.08
Rhythm interpretation: Sinus bradycardia ventricular bigeminy

Strip 13.105
Rhythm: Regular
Rate: 84
P wave: P wave after the QRS
PR interval: N/A
QRS complex: 0.14
Rhythm interpretation: Accelerated junctional

Strip 13.106
Rhythm: Irregular
Rate: 250
P wave: None
PR interval: N/A
QRS complex: Wide
Rhythm interpretation: Ventricular tachycardia

Strip 13.107
Rhythm: Irregular
Rate: 70
P wave: Sinus in a few beats
PR interval: Varies 0.12-0.16
QRS complex: 0.08
Rhythm interpretation: 2 sinus beats, premature junctional complex, 2 sinus beats, premature ventricular contraction, 1 sinus beat

Strip 13.108
Rhythm: Regular
Rate: 125
P wave: P wave in the T wave
PR interval: N/A
QRS complex: 0.08
Rhythm interpretation: Sinus tachycardia with 1 premature ventricular contraction

Strip 13.109
Rhythm: Irregular
Rate: 70 paced converting to a rate of 250
P wave: None
PR interval: N/A
QRS complex: Wide
Rhythm interpretation: Ventrical paced with R-on-T phenomenon ventricular tachycardia

Strip 13.110
Rhythm: Irregular
Rate: 0
P wave: 0
PR interval: 0
QRS complex: 0
Rhythm interpretation: Asystole with 1 agonal beat

Strip 13.111
Rhythm: Regular–Irregular
Rate: 113
P wave: Sinus
PR interval: 0.16
QRS complex: 0.06
Rhythm interpretation: Sinus tachycardia with ventricular quadreminy

Strip 13.112
Rhythm: Irregular
Rate: 84-150
P wave: Sinus
PR interval: 0.12
QRS complex: Notched 0.12
Rhythm interpretation: Normal sinus rhythm with bundle branch block and 6 beat run of ventricular tachycardia

Strip 13.113
Rhythm: Regular
Rate: 50
P wave: 2 P waves for every QRS
PR interval: 0.20
QRS complex: 0.10
Rhythm interpretation: 2nd degree type II with 2:1 conduction, 1 premature ventricular contraction after the 5th complex

Strip 13.114
Rhythm: Irregular
Rate: 250
P wave: 0
PR interval: 0
QRS complex: 0
Rhythm interpretation: Ventricular tachycardia with a pacemaker programmed with an antitachyarrythmia function.

Strip 13.115
AV interval rate: 85
Chamber paced: Ventricular
Sensing: Appropriately
Capture: 100%
Pacing interpretation: Sensing and capturing appropriately, ventricular bigeminy

Strip 13.116
AV interval rate: 75
Chamber paced: Ventricular
Sensing: Appropriately
Capture: 100%
Pacing interpretation: 4 ventricular-paced beats, 1 pseudofusion beat, 3 intrinsic beats, 2 paced beats

Strip 13.117
AV interval rate: 65
Chamber paced: Atrial
Sensing: Appropriately
Capture: 100%
Pacing interpretation: Sensing and capturing appropriately

Strip 13.118
AV interval rate: 75
Chamber paced: Atrial
Sensing: Appropriately
Capture: 100%
Pacing interpretation: Sensing and capturing appropriately

Strip 13.119
AV interval rate: 220
Chamber paced: 0
Sensing: 0
Capture: 0
Pacing interpretation: Ventricular tachycardia with a pacemaker attempting to break with its antitachyarrhythmia function

Strip 13.120
AV interval rate: 100
Chamber paced: Ventricular
Sensing: No
Capture: Yes
Pacing interpretation: 4 paced beats, 2 intrinsic beats, inappropriate sensed spike on 8th beat, 1 paced beat, R-on-T going into a ventricular tachycardia

Strip 13.121
AV interval rate: 125
Chamber paced: Dual
Sensing: Yes
Capture: Yes
Pacing interpretation: 10 ventricular-paced beats, 1 atrioventicular-paced beat, 6 ventricular-paced beats

Strip 13.122
AV interval rate: 75
Chamber paced: Ventricular
Sensing: Yes
Capture: Yes
Pacing interpretation: 1 ventricular-paced beat, 1 intrinsic beat, 4 more ventricular-paced beats, 1 intrinsic beat, 3 ventricular-paced beats

Strip 13.123
AV interval rate: 65
Chamber paced: Atrial
Sensing: Yes
Capture: Yes
Pacing interpretation: 100% atria paced

Strip 13.124
AV interval rate: 63 (intrinsic)
Chamber paced: 0
Sensing: 0
Capture: 0
Pacing interpretation: Atrial flutter

Strip 13.125
AV interval rate: 100 (intrinsic)
Chamber paced: 0
Sensing: 0
Capture: 0
Pacing interpretation: Controlled atrial fibrillation

Strip 13.126
AV interval rate: 60
Chamber paced: Ventricular
Sensing: Yes
Capture: Yes
Pacing interpretation: 100% ventricle paced

Strip 13.127
AV interval rate: 88
Chamber paced: Ventricular
Sensing: Yes
Capture: Yes
Pacing interpretation: 100% ventricle paced

Strip 13.128
AV interval rate: 56
Chamber paced: Ventricular
Sensing: Yes
Capture: Yes
Pacing interpretation: 1 intrinsic beat, 3 ventricular-paced beats, 1 intrinsic beat

Strip 13.129
AV interval rate: Intrinsic rate 60
Chamber paced: Ventricular
Sensing: Yes
Capture: Yes
Pacing interpretation: 4 intrinsic beats, 1 ventricular-paced beat, 3 intrinsic beats, 1 ventricular-paced beat, 2 intrinsic beats

Strip 13.130
AV interval rate: 75
Chamber paced: Ventricular
Sensing: No
Capture: No
Pacing interpretation: Complete heart block, a failure to capture and not sensing intrinsic activity

Strip 13.131
AV interval rate:
Chamber paced: Ventricular
Sensing: Yes
Capture: Yes
Pacing interpretation: 6 intrinsic beats, 1 ventricular-paced beat, 4 intrinsic beats

INDEX